YOUR KIDNEY/MY KIDNEY

WRITTEN AND RESEARCHED
BY
DONNA-MARIE H. POLLARD

Batax Museum Publishing
2051 Wheeler Lane
Jacksonville, FL 32259

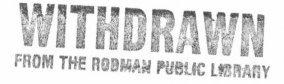

The names of the medical facilities, persons, and characters in this book are fictitious, and any resemblance to actual medical facilities, persons, or characters, living or dead, is purely coincidental.

Library of Congress Cataloging-in-Publication Data
(Prepared by Pollard, Donna-Marie H.)

Your Kidney/My Kidney / Written and Researched by
Donna-Marie H. Pollard

p. cm.
Includes bibliographical references, glossary of
medical terms and index.
 ISBN:0-9629759-0-7 (v. 1): $19.95
 First Printing 2001
 I. Title.

DEDICATION

This book is dedicated to the memory of Lina Maria Fierro, Aida Sylvia Pollard, Manuel Innocente Fierro, and Michael Anthony Pollard.

and

To my sister Joanne for her unfailing and unconditional love and support, for being my very best friend, and giving me the greatest gift that I have ever received, a kidney.

TABLE OF CONTENTS

CONTENTS (CONT'D)

FOREWORD

For centuries, mankind has sought to save afflicted people from failure of vital organs, and the thought of organ replacement has been in the realm of either the mythical or superstitious. As the twentieth century closes, however, we have learned the skills to save and renew the lives of many patients who otherwise would die without an organ transplant. Liver, heart, and lung transplantation are now undertaken when no other form of treatment can save the patient. Kidney, pancreas, and intestinal transplantation are carried out when it is determined that the transplanted organ will render optimum treatment for the patient having kidney failure, severe diabetes, or severe malnutrition. The evolution of medicines which maintain transplanted organs has assured a positive outcome of organ transplantation for the vast majority of patients. Unfortunately, the shortage of willing organ donors still dooms many persons, who could benefit by an organ transplant.

Your Kidney/My Kidney is a remarkable story about one person's varied experiences in living with kidney failure. Donna Pollard recounts in considerable detail what the change from seemingly good and stable health to the need for an organ transplant was like. She is able to carry the reader on her journey, even when medical, surgical, and medication complications appear to be the order of the day.

Especially for patients with kidney failure, Your Kidney/My Kidney deals with many familiar steps in dialysis and transplant areas. For patients having failure of other organs, Your Kidney/My Kidney may also be instructive as the final common pathways of organ transplantation are similar for most organ transplant recipients. Details in the glossary and appendix also may be of great assistance to many who follow Donna Pollard's course and have an interest in learning more about organ failure, organ donation, and transplantation.

Your Kidney/My Kidney brings many of the real life patient issues forward. Enjoy and learn.

Thomas G. Peters, M.D.
Jacksonville, Florida

ACKNOWLEDGEMENTS

Mere words are not sufficient to express my gratitude to:

- My sister Joanne-Marie, my family, and friends Nancy, Jose, Barbara, Rosalia, Debbie, Greg, Katherine, Pam, Suzie, Tracy, Mike, Joe, Hope and Cynthia for their love and support.
- The "Blue People" from the laboratory who are too numerous to mention for fear of exclusion.
- Rebecca Reams, for her tirelessness in attending to my every need.
- The health care providers including my transplant team, whom I especially recognize and credit for saving my life.
- David Anthony Vernoia, for his superb care after my numerous surgeries, for making me laugh with his unique sense of humor, but most importantly, for simply being there.

Foreword
- Thomas G. Peters, M.D.

Reviewers
- Hope Greig, MSH, MT(ASCP)SC
- Ellen W. Bryan, LPN, Retired
- Suzanne Pepper, RN, CCRN
- George Walker, RN, BSN, CCRN

Editor
- Erma Torsiello

Computers
- Deanna Treloar, for the loan of her computer to accomplish the first draft of this book.
- David Reams, for his help with my many computer needs.

Cover Design, Illustrations & Typesetting
- Joanne-Marie Pollard

Afterword
- Ellen W. Bryan

Finally, thanks to my cockatiel, Jake, my ever faithful and loving companion for never failing to say to me the one word he knows, **"Hello!"**

DISCLAIMER

The publisher and author are not engaged in rendering medical services and/or advice. This book is designed to provide information relative to the subject matter covered. It is sold with the understanding that the publisher and author are not engaged in rendering medical services. If medical expert assistance is required, the services of a competent professional should be sought.

The purpose of this book is to educate, and inspire. The author and Batax Museum Publishing shall have neither liability nor responsibility to any person or entity with respect to any information taken or used or alleged to be taken or used out of context from this book.

Every effort has been made to make the information presented in this book as accurate as possible. However, there may be mistakes both typographical or in content. The information contained in this book is a detailed and chronological account of one person's experiences while battling kidney disease. It is meant to share with the reader possible events or side effects that a kidney transplant patient may experience.

If you do not wish to be bound by the above, you may return this book to the publisher for a full refund.

ABOUT THE AUTHOR

As therapy, during my hemodialysis treatments, I began making a chronological record of the symptoms and progression of my disease, Polycystic Kidney Disease (PKD). This record began from the time I was diagnosed with PKD to the present.

In the interest of educating myself, I interviewed several End-Stage Renal Disease (ESRD), dialysis, and transplant patients. Apart from the notes I took during these interviews, I read all materials available to me and went to my regularly scheduled appointments with my nephrologist, armed with a list of questions.

The result was that I managed to gather a wealth of information, and as this information grew, my stack of handwritten pages grew in proportion. With tongue in cheek, I titled my writings "Things Your Doctors Don't Tell You." While reading my notes, I was struck by the feeling that I should share this valuable information with other patients who find themselves in a similar situation.

Not many patients are fortunate enough to have had access to all the information I did, and most are so ill they do not have the energy to expend toward information gathering. The challenge, as I saw it, was how to disseminate this information in such a way that it would benefit other patients and, hopefully, uplift and inspire. I also felt that perhaps kidney patients everywhere needed a champion. Why not me?! I began to seriously organize my notes. This book is the result.

As I share my story, I will delve into the psyche of the typical kidney patient and explain the changes which take place in their lives. I talk openly about my transplant and subsequent loss of the graft and the ensuing anger. I hope to demonstrate to other kidney patients that many of the emotions and thoughts that plague them are, in fact, normal stages of the process that we, as kidney patients, all go through: shock, denial, anger, depression, low self-esteem and morale, desire to die, acceptance, then finally, hopefully, change of behavior.

My story begins about the time I was thirteen years of age, when one of my mother's older sisters, Lina, died of complete renal failure and other complications.

Four years later my mother, Aida, also died from complete renal failure at the age of thirty-seven. One year later, my mother's youngest brother, Manuel, also succumbed to complete renal failure at the age of thirty-five. After the third death occurred, we concluded that this was no coincidence and believed that our family ranks were being depleted by a kidney disease that was genetic in nature and had an adult onset.

One week after my younger brother Michael Anthony was diagnosed with kidney disease, I too was diagnosed with kidney disease by my physician in Colorado. After several days of dealing with this fact, I began considering my options. I also needed time to find the strength and the right words to break the news to my family, especially my father. After eighteen months of being on hemodialysis, Michael developed complications and died on June 8, 1993 at the age of 31. Death was becoming a familiar companion.

Over the span of twenty-seven years, during which time the first three deaths occurred, we lived on the two-island, English-speaking nation, Trinidad & Tobago in that part of the Caribbean known as the West Indies. Because the islands had limited medical resources, my relatives did not have the same chance for survival that I had. By the time their kidney disease was discovered, their kidney function had already deteriorated to the point of zero function. Little was known about kidney diseases at that time in the Caribbean. There were no dialysis machines or kidney transplant programs. There was also a matter of finances. We simply waited for them to die.

By the time Michael was diagnosed with kidney disease in October of 1991, there were several dialysis centers on the island, and a transplant program was in the process of being established. Sadly, Michael died before the government of Trinidad & Tobago decided to fund his kidney transplant. I was very fortunate that my kidney disease was diagnosed in the United States, so my chances for survival were greatly increased.

Prior to the diagnosis of my kidney disease at the age of 35, I had led a normal, happy life, filled with a wide variety of activities. I was enrolled in college and looking forward to a bright future. However, following this diagnosis, my life changed drastically. I went from a life filled with activities and expectations to a stationary existence with nothing but time to reflect.

CHAPTER ONE

TIAs, THE FIRST SIGN OF TROUBLE

"The body is a sacred garment. It's your first and last garment; it is what you enter life in and what you depart life with, and it should be treated with honor."
-Martha Graham

Arriving at my diagnosis was not as straight forward as one would suppose. In actuality, in took several years for my disease to be diagnosed. It all began with frequent migraine headaches and symptoms of hypertension (high blood pressure), which eventually became debilitating. Dr. Harold Saunders, my primary care physician at the time, believed that my blood pressure could be controlled through diet. For me, this meant abstinence from all forms of sodium and foods high in sodium content.

Not many months had gone by when Dr. Saunders and I both realized that diet was not the answer to controlling my physical ailments. Dr. Saunders recommended various antihypertensive and diuretic (water pill) medications on a trial and error basis. These medications caused me to have dry mouth and eyes. The dry eyes proved to be horrendous for me as a contact lens wearer. The medications also produced an allergic type of reaction in the form of a rash. None of the medications provided any relief from my migraine headaches.

Rushing off to work one morning, I forgot to take my blood pressure medication. It was not until that evening when I realized I had not experienced a headache all day.

The following day, I took my medication and I again experienced a migraine headache. I decided to discontinue my medication for several days to see what effect this would have. The result was no migraine headaches on those medication-free days. When I visited Dr. Saunders at his office for a blood pressure check, we discovered that my blood pressure was normal. He felt it was time to discontinue the medications.

Being the high energy person that I have always been, I was happy to be free of the rigorous constraints resulting from the medications. I was once again able to continue my church activities and work a forty-hour work week. Even with the constraints, I had still managed to find time to go to movies, attend my favorite plays and concerts, do some hiking and travelling, and still walk three miles every day.

Off and on, I was still plagued with high blood pressure and migraine headaches. At each of my monthly visits with Dr. Saunders, he would again institute another hypertensive on a trial and error basis. Once my blood pressure and headaches were under control, we would again discontinue the medication. Something was still wrong; my headaches kept reoccurring. It was apparent by this time that Dr. Saunders did not know what to do. He believed my high blood pressure could have been caused by any number of a wide variety of ailments. Living in the Mile High City, Denver, Colorado with its high altitude was suspected to be the culprit. I believed we were treating my symptoms and not getting to the root of my problem. Tests were ordered but were inconclusive. My kidney function tests were elevated, such as, blood urea nitrogen [(BUN) (the urea concentration of blood or serum stated in terms of nitrogen content] and Creatinine (the end product of creatine metabolism). Creatine is released into the blood stream during the aerobic phase of muscle contraction, e.g., aerobic exercise.

I was concerned about the test results, but Dr. Saunders did not seem to think they were highly significant, and no further tests were ordered. In retrospect, I realize now that this was the most positive indication that I had a kidney disease.

My sister, Joanne, arrived the same day my husband, Douglas, left for a three-month work assignment in Southern California. While Joanne and I were watching television one evening, my next symptom made its appearance.

There seemed to be a pulsatile swishing in my right ear which I interpreted as the sound of heavy breathing. I told Joanne that I could not believe how loudly her dog was breathing and proceeded to chase poor Jitzu out of the room.

Though Jitzu was no longer in the room with us, I could still hear the "breathing." I realized then that the sound was in sync with my heartbeat and made a mental note to telephone Dr. Saunders about this new development the following morning.

Two days later, I began having mild strokes. One of these episodes caused the entire left side of my body to become completely numb as I was driving home from work one afternoon. Luckily, I had the presence of mind not to panic. My only thought at the time was to arrive home safely and call my doctor. Upon arriving home, I telephoned Dr. Saunders, only to be told that he was not available but that I could speak to his associate. His associate reviewed my chart, telephoned me at home, and we proceeded to play twenty questions. One-half hour into the question and answer session, he asked if my left side was still numb. I responded that it was subsiding and that feeling was returning in my left hand and arm. Because the duration of the numbness was so short, he felt that these symptoms, while not very common, were nothing more than a "strange neurological effect brought on by my migraine headaches," and he ended our conversation by telling me not to worry.

During the following five days I would have a total of six mild strokes. Later, I learned they were actually transient ischemic attacks [(TIAs) (stroke-like symptoms of short duration]. As a result of the TIAs, I developed a limp. By the end of each day, I was exhausted from the effort of controlling the quiver in my right hip and leg. I also began having problems controlling my hands. This created a very difficult situation, as part of my responsibilities at work included a significant amount of typing.

On the morning of the fifth day, I found myself stopping more frequently to massage my hands, hoping that feeling and control would return. Also, I developed a migraine of such proportion that I could barely function. It felt as though the entire right side of my face would explode and a red hot needle was piercing through my right eye to the back of my skull. In an attempt to control the pain, I consumed so many pain killers that only fear of an overdose prevented my taking more.

I developed a very bad case of dry mouth and left my desk in search of a drink of water. On the return trip to my desk I could feel both my legs going numb. The numbness was slowly creeping upward and had achieved waist level. All I could think of at the time was getting to my desk to call my doctor. It occurred to me that I should use the wall for support. In the event I should fall, I would slide down the wall to the floor, and avoid falling forward and injuring my head.

William Bradley, my supervisor, saw me in the hallway and asked if I was alright, to which I replied, "No, I cannot feel my legs." William asked Kyle Anderson, a co-worker, to get me a chair while William supported me in an upright position by my arms. William and Kyle quickly wheeled me back to my desk. By this time my entire body, including my face, felt numb. I could no longer hold my head erect, my tongue felt as though it were three times its normal size, and I could not speak clearly. I motioned for Amy Garrett, our department secretary, to retrieve my address book from my handbag. I managed to find Dr. Saunders' name and number as I fumbled through the pages under the "S's."

Dr. Saunders said that I should wait twenty or thirty minutes and if the numbness subsided during that time, I had nothing to worry about. If, on the other hand, it did not subside, I should present myself at his office. Incensed, William told Amy to call Dr. Saunders again, and inform him that I was in fact on my way to his office.

Richard Borelli, another co-worker, helped me into his car, then proceeded to break the sound barrier getting me to Dr. Saunders' office. Upon arrival, Dr. Saunders discovered that my blood pressure was an astronomical 250/150 mm/Hg! (Normal range 120/80 mm/Hg). He recommended that I be admitted to St. Bridget's Hospital immediately. "I do not have time for this, right now," I said. Little did I know my body had other plans for me.

I was barely able to stand. What a sight we were, Richard and I both struggling to remove my jewelry in the hospital parking lot. Richard carried the paperwork in one hand and steadied me with the other. Upon reaching the entrance, I ceremoniously placed all my jewelry in Richard's hand with the words, "Lose it and die." He faithfully promised to give the precious treasures to my sister, so his life would not be in jeopardy.

By this time, my head kept falling from one side to the other, as I struggled to hold it erect. As I was wearing my sunglasses at the time, I began bobbing and weaving my head, and I chidingly asked Richard how he liked my "rock star" impression. Richard practically collapsed with laughter. He could not believe that I was making jokes under the circumstances.

Upon admission, I was immediately taken in a wheelchair to a private room and was given two Extra Strength Tylenol® and 80 mg of Inderal® to control my headache and blood pressure. I had just donned my hospital gown when a technician swept into my room wheeling her equipment to perform an Electrocardiogram (ECG). The ECG only took a few minutes to perform. It involved the strategic placement of several leads to my chest and legs. These leads produced a graphic record on paper of the electrical variations in action of my heart muscles.

A Computed Axial Tomography (CAT) scan was also performed. The actual machine was like a donut with a hole in the center. This particular test was painless. I was placed on a narrow sort of table which slid back and forth through the hole in the center of the machine. It was just a matter of lying motionless and holding my breath, as the CAT scan machine took a series of x-rays of my head and neck. These x-rays were taken as though my head and neck were in consecutive slices approximately 5-7 microns thin. There were flashing lights, a humming sound as the x-rays were taken, and a warning not to look directly at the red light of the laser. Because these test results were normal and revealed nothing of my true condition, I remained afraid and confused.

I telephoned my sister and my visiting and home teachers from church. They all arrived at the hospital shortly thereafter to administer to my emotional and spiritual needs. With these needs met, I settled in for the night and reflected on the events of the day.

CHAPTER TWO

MY FIRST MRI, AND ANGIOGRAM

> *"The first wealth is health."*
> -Ralph Waldo Emerson

I had a difficult time living within the confines of my altered, slower-paced lifestyle. I was unable to let go of what I saw as my "responsibilities." From my hospital bed, I continued to arrange, confirm, and solicit commitments from those who promised to assist me with my current church-related projects.

While this drama was unfolding in Colorado, my husband was still working in Southern California, and Joanne and I spent most of our time at home because of my health situation. Douglas was only allowed one weekend off every two weeks, during which time he would come home. Other than those rare weekends, my contact with him was limited to two phone calls a day. My sister became my sole source of support. It seemed that her visit was coordinated by a higher source, a source that I would come to depend on and literally trust my very being, that source being my Heavenly Father.

The following morning after my admission to the hospital, my sister was helping me bathe when a female physician entered my room. Apparently, Dr. Saunders had requested a neurological consultation from Dr. Frances Farnsworth. She put me through some of the most grueling tests during the ensuing 48 hours.

The first of these tests was a spinal tap (procedure by which spinal fluid is obtained for analysis) which she performed herself. Dr. Farnsworth anesthetized the site for insertion of the needle by injecting a quantity of Lidocaine®. After the stinging subsided I felt a little pressure as a long needle was inserted into my spine.

Dr. Farnsworth then pulled back on the plunger of the syringe and aspirated a quantity of spinal fluid for analysis. She said the good news was that visually my spinal fluid was clear. There was no obvious sign of bleeding or infection. The bad news was, after the procedure I had to lie perfectly still for six to eight hours to prevent headaches. That day several scans and ultrasounds were also performed. The ultrasound revealed decreased right internal carotid artery (ICA) flow, which Dr. Farnsworth suspected was caused by a blockage. Following this discovery, I was shuttled in an ambulance during a snow storm, to St. Mary's Hospital.

The ride in the ambulance was not what I expected. I was sitting in a wheelchair which was secured to the floor of the ambulance. Once strapped in, several warm blankets were wrapped around me to keep me warm. I felt like a caterpillar in a cocoon. I had the impression that when patients traveled by ambulance they were lying down, not seated. I did not have the pleasure of lying down, nor did the driver use the siren. I felt as though I was cheated of the opportunity to enjoy the full experience. Well, I thought, at least I got to enjoy the snow fall with its huge, fluffy snowflakes.

Upon arriving at St. Mary's Hospital, I was taken away to have an magnetic resonance imaging (MRI) study performed. The test itself is not painful. It is only uncomfortable for patients who are large in stature or afflicted with claustrophobia. I never knew that I was claustrophobic until that day.

My forehead was strapped down with Velcro® to keep my head immobile and my arms were strapped at my sides to keep them from falling off the very narrow gurney-type of bed, which protruded from the MRI machine. A neurovascular head koil was pulled down over my face. The table began moving slowly. I was entering the machine head first into what appeared to be a very small, stark white, cylindrical tunnel. Once in the machine, little lights started blinking and a very loud clanging began. I was not sure what was happening to me. I only knew that my heart was beating wildly.

My heart beat faster and faster, until I thought it would leap from my chest. I felt my blood pressure rising, and my temples felt as though they would explode. My head ached horribly and my breathing became shallow and erratic. I began panting like a puppy. I was experiencing an anxiety attack and felt as though the cold, clammy, hand of fear had reached out and touched my heart, mind and very soul. My imagination was rampant.

I imagined I was experiencing how it felt to be buried alive. I began hollering, "I cannot do this, take me out of here!" I had never felt so panic-stricken before. I felt foolish. How could I be so afraid of a test which did not involve any pain? I could feel my fear subsiding as I was being taken out of the machine, and the faces of the nurses in attendance came into view. The supervisor was summoned.

Her face bore a very sympathetic expression as she explained to me that I had a very common reaction experienced by many patients. Because I would not allow myself to be placed in the machine again, the nurse administered a quantity of Valium intravenously. I told the technicians that it was a pity they did not have a way to pipe music into the MRI machine. It would take the patient's mind off the cramptness and the noise produced by the MRI machine. I was surprised when headphones were produced and placed on my head, and as if by magic, I began to hear the familiar strains of the music of my favorite radio station 102.9 FM. A washcloth was placed over my eyes, to prevent me from opening them. I was strapped in and we began the test again. All I remember was asking someone to talk to me as I was in the MRI machine. The next time I opened my eyes the procedure was over. I must have been traveling in the wonderful world of Valium® or the Valley of The Dolls.

The nurses decided not to remove the intravenous catheter (IV) in the event I required further testing. Much to my chagrin, one hour later Dr. Farnsworth advised me that based on the results of the MRI, a right carotid angiogram was indicated. As I signed the appropriate consent forms, I told Dr. Farnsworth that I was prepared to endure whatever was required, as long as she deemed it absolutely necessary for the diagnosis of my health problem.

Dr. Stanley Baxter, the physician designated to perform the angiogram, spent fifteen minutes explaining what he saw on my MRI. He saw several abnormalities in my brain and, to the best of his knowledge, he believed that I had experienced seven to ten strokes. Dr. Baxter further stated that it was suspected that I had sustained some damage to one of the arteries leading to my brain. The carotid angiograms would reveal the precise location of the damage. Additional medication was administered and I was wheeled into an Operating Room (OR) to have the angiogram performed. I did not believe at the time that enough medication was administered before or after the procedure.

I felt the scalpel cut into my right groin. I, at once, felt very warm liquid flowing down my genital area and over my right thigh. I realized that this warm liquid could only be my own blood. It was terrifying! The catheter which was white, almost thread-like, was inserted in my right femoral artery. Then, dye at high pressure was shot from what looked like a space-aged ray gun through the catheter and up to my brain.

Although I was warned with a "Here it comes," it still did not prepare me for the pain and burning that accompanied the dye. It was shot first up the right side and then the left side of my brain. During the seconds that seemed like hours of pain and burning, I had to remain completely motionless. I had to hold my breath and was not allowed even so much as a grimace while the x-rays were being taken. Of all the tests that were performed during the first forty-eight hours of my hospitalization, the angiogram was the most physically stressful and painful.

Once the test was completed, one of the nurses had to apply direct pressure to the wound in my right groin for fifteen minutes, using the full force of his weight. The pain was the worst I had ever experienced and seemed to last an eternity.

As the nurse counted down the number of minutes left to apply pressure, I became very cold, and felt as though I was going into shock because my body began to shake uncontrollably on the operating table. I asked for some more medication and was given several additional injections of Lidocaine® directly into my right groin. It had no effect whatsoever and the pain continued to the point of delirium.

Once the fifteen minutes were up, the pain persisted. I was wheeled into the Intensive Care Unit (ICU) where a nurse was assigned to stay with me. I asked if there was anything she could do to control the pain. I felt that I was losing control, and knew that crying would only intensify the headache I was already experiencing.

The nurse excused herself and hurried back with a plastic bag containing several ice cubes. She further wrapped the bag in a washcloth and placed it on my right groin.

The initial weight of the ice on my groin actually intensified the pain. I prayed that I would faint! No such luck! I gritted my teeth and, in a few minutes, miraculously, the pain subsided. I could finally rest and maybe even sleep. I was exhausted. I felt physically, emotionally, and mentally drained, as though I had scrubbed the entire floor of the Smithsonian Museum on my knees with a tooth-brush. Several hours later, I was removed from the ICU and prepared for shuttle back to my room at St. Bridget's Hospital.

The ambulance this time was manned by very young paramedics, one male, and one female. This time I got to lie down! Ah! Life was good I thought, as I lay strapped in listening to the sound of the siren. It was the high point of my day. I felt as though a childhood dream had been fulfilled. Once we cleared the traffic, the siren was turned off which allowed for conversation with the paramedics. The only discomfort I experienced occurred when the ambulance drove over a bump or pothole.

CHAPTER THREE

CAUSE OF TIAs DIAGNOSED

> *"There is a limit to the best of health: disease
> is always a near neighbor."*
>
> **-AESCHYLUS, Agamemnon**

Once I arrived at St. Bridget's, I was placed in the ICU and as I waited for Dr. Farnsworth to arrive, I had a few minutes to reflect.

I thought about Joanne and the fact that she was not having much of a visit. She divided her time between taking care of the four dogs that we owned between us at the townhome and spending a great portion of the day with me at the hospital. I resolved to make it up to her once I was released and recuperated.

Dr. Farnsworth arrived later that evening and proceeded with pen and paper to draw and describe what the angiogram had revealed. Apparently, my right carotid artery, which is to the front and side of my neck, consists of three layers. The inner most layer had disconnected from the other layers of the artery. While disconnecting, some bleeding had occurred which in turn had formed a clot. This clot caused a constriction of the lumen (the innermost layer) of the artery. The blood, coursing through the artery, was obliged to force its way through the narrowed portion of vessel. This caused the pulsatile swishing sound (rhythmic expansion of an artery which may be felt with the finger) or bruit (the human pulse) I heard in my right ear.

Each time the blood forced its way through the narrowed vessel, bits of blood clot were being dislodged and carried up to my brain. The network of vessels became smaller and smaller the further they travelled away from a major artery. The tiny blood clots travelled along until they encountered thread-like vessels (capillaries) through which they could not flow, causing blockages. These blockages caused an insufficient supply of oxygen to areas of my brain, producing TIAs. This was the culprit and cause of all the numbness and headaches.

Although the last forty-eight hours were gruelling, it was a relief to finally have a diagnosis and know my options. I spent the next two days in the ICU and was not allowed to do anything unaided. That was very difficult for me to endure and I became very restless. I asked one of the nurses to wash and blow dry my hair. She did and I felt better at once. I very slowly brushed my teeth then began the arduous process of applying make-up. Approximately one hour had elapsed before I completed the task.

At one point, I looked up and noticed that I had an audience. One of the nurses came over and said that never before had she seen anyone apply make-up while in the ICU. She asked whether I was fully aware of the gravity of my situation. I responded that I knew and understood only too well. I further explained that I dealt with my problems with humor and tried to behave in as normal a fashion as possible. Since I seldom have an audience, I took advantage of the situation and took a bow, to which I received a round of applause. Of course, we kept it all at a dull roar.

Once out of the ICU, I had a steady stream of visitors. I was surprised that I knew so many people considering that I had only lived in Littleton, Colorado, for two and a half years. Everyone came bearing gifts, but I especially appreciated the well wishes, prayers, and seeing their smiling faces. I was fortunate to be in a large room, because this allowed for the addition of an extra table to accommodate all the bouquets and cards I received.

It was a most difficult time in my life, but it was also one of the most joyful experiences, knowing that I had touched so many lives. It was wonderful to know that there were still many people in this world who care about others. I felt blessed! I still needed a miracle, however. If the inner lining of my right carotid artery would not re-adhere with the current course of anticoagulation therapy (blood thinner), I would require surgery.

A portion of artery would be removed from another area of my body and used as a graft to replace the affected portion of artery in my neck. My progress during the following days would determine whether or not surgery would be required.

The combination of anticoagulant and antihypertensive medications lowered my blood pressure to such a degree that I could not stand without fainting. The dosage of antihypertensives was reduced and immediately saline was added to my IV to raise my blood pressure to an acceptable level.

I prayed more fervently than ever, asking for strength to overcome my illness and to endure whatever was to come. I started to grow in strength. My kidney function tests were beginning to improve and my blood pressure was under control. My fear was replaced with a sense of peace and the actual belief that I would have a full recovery. Several days later, I was told that my doctors were so pleased with my progress that I would be released. The night before I was due to be released, I experienced what was the worst of the TIAs. I also experienced problems swallowing and breathing. Needless to say, my stay in the hospital was extended. By this time, I had grown so accustomed to having my blood pressure checked all though the night, that I would automatically extend my arm without opening my eyes each time I heard the nurse approaching.

After another battery of tests, a mass was discovered in my liver, which I was told was benign. Cysts were found in my kidneys. I was told that it is very common to have cysts without any specific significance in various parts of the body. The cysts on x-ray were benign-appearing, consequently, they were not taken into account. A nephrologist came to see me while I was in the hospital. He told me that my kidney function tests had returned to normal and there was no need for follow-up. A right carotid ultrasound was performed, and the inner lining of the artery was revealed to be almost completely re-adhered. Surgical repair was not indicated. I was to continue with my regimen of Coumadin® (oral anticoagulant/blood thinner) and have a repeat right carotid angiogram in three months.

The ultrasound was performed by applying heated gel to the right side of my neck, which allowed the transducer to slide easily over the area. With the use of ultrasounds, which produced ultrasonic echoes, a photographic image was produced of the underlying structures.

At my place of employment I had accumulated five weeks of extended leave with pay and I was strongly encouraged to take it. I had to agree. I was very weak and needed the time to recuperate and build my strength. I was also having problems with my short-term memory and speech. I would have a clear image of the specific word I wanted to say, but by the time the word made its way to my mouth, it was translated into something quite different. It was confusing. I was told that these symptoms were sometimes experienced by patients on anticoagulation therapy and the classic aftermath of a stroke or TIA.

Follow-up blood work was being performed, especially to monitor my prothrombin time (PT) and partial thromboplastin time (PTT). After each blood drawing, ice was placed on my antecubital fossa (bend in the arm opposite the elbow) for 20 minutes to promote clotting. I could not use a razor to shave, and I kept out of the kitchen to avoid cutting myself. With the level of anticoagulants in my system, if I were to sustain a cut, my blood simply would not clot. My imagination, however, was not impaired. I could envision the headlines, "Woman Survives Strokes But Bleeds To Death From Paper Cut." Could you imagine a more senseless way to die? I wanted to live long and die an old woman, who annoys other motorists, by leaving my turn signal on for miles.

During my convalescence, a steady stream of visitors continued to visit my home and many of my friends from church brought meals so my sister and I would not have to concern ourselves with cooking. It was rough, but we managed.

On one of my return visits to Dr. Saunders, I asked if it was necessary to follow-up with the nephrologist as well as the neurologist. I was told that follow-up with my neurologist was necessary, but not with the nephrologist because my kidney function tests were normal and the few cysts found in my kidneys were thought to be benign-appearing, and not significant.

During this time I was not allowed to exercise, and my physical activity consisted of walking up and down stairs, very slowly. I became tired with very little exertion and was advised to get as much bed rest as possible. As a result of this inertia, I began gaining weight. I was in agony! Prior to becoming ill, I had managed to turn my three-mile walks into six-mile walks as often as I could manage it. I thoroughly enjoyed being on the go.

CHAPTER FOUR

POLYCYSTIC KIDNEY DISEASE

"One loses many laughs by not laughing at oneself."

-Sara Jeannette Duncan

Douglas was now back home and Joanne was in Canoga Park, Southern California visiting relatives. Not only did I have to deal with the trauma of being separated from my sister, but I also had to face the impending repeat angiogram.

By now, I had returned to work and attempted to pick up where I left off. I did not have the same energy level I had before. My tragic events had taken its toll and I came to the realization that it would take a long time for me to fully recover.

The thought that I had to have a repeat right carotid angiogram in two months was constantly with me. The day that I had dreaded for so long finally arrived, and I was once again admitted to the hospital. I prayed that the impending repeat procedure would not be as painful as the last.

Dr. Baxter, the physician who performed the original angiogram would also be performing the second angiogram. My neurologist felt that I would be more comfortable with a familiar face. It also helped that I was given a quantity of Valium® intravenously. Valium® created a state of calm causing all my anxieties to disappear. I would not care what was done to me if a sufficient quantity was administered. Valium®! The wonder drug! Ask for it by name!

The repeat angiogram was a much better experience than the first. I did not feel the initial incision, and the entire procedure was pain free. I even dozed on and off through the procedure. During my lucid moments, I did not seem to mind the fact that both the catheter and the physician's gloves were blood stained.

Once the procedure was completed, I slept as much as I could, while waiting for Douglas to take me home. My recovery time was much shorter than that of the first angiogram. Initially, it took me three days before I could walk upright. This time, I could walk upright almost immediately, although I still could not climb stairs for at least twenty-four hours.

The angiogram revealed that the inner lining of my right carotid artery had completely re-adhered. Surgery would definitely not be indicated. I did, however, have to control my blood pressure at all cost because of beading/bulging of the artery. Again I felt lucky because many patients have such severe beading or bulging, that their carotid arteries have the appearance of a string of pearls and require surgery. It seemed to me that I was living a charmed life. I had a lot to be thankful for.

Three months later my neurologist was pleased with my progress and the anticoagulants were discontinued. My blood pressure was also normal and Dr. Saunders discontinued the antihypertensives.

My activity level was still very low. It was still too soon to resume my walks and I had been released from my church calling. I was forced to participate in gentler pursuits, such as reading, cross stitching, and the like.

I had almost forgotten my ordeal until one year later, when I began experiencing migraine headaches again, and in the same right side of my face. Back I went to Dr. Saunders and he discovered that my blood pressure had risen to an unacceptable level and needed to be controlled. We, again, began a trial of several different types of antihypertensives. Some caused severe nausea, others headaches, and yet others were too strong and lowered my blood pressure to an unacceptably low level, so low as to impede activity.

After a period of several weeks I had experienced enough pain and decided to telephone Dr. Farnsworth and ask for her help. I shared with her the fact that I was unsatisfied with my medical care and that I was once again hypertensive and experiencing migraine headaches.

I asked her to recommend a good primary care physician. She recommended a female internist by the name of Dr. Cheryl Casey. I liked Dr. Casey instantly. She was very efficient, capable, caring, and professional. Within fifteen minutes of speaking to me, she suspected that I had a type of kidney disease given my family history, but diagnosis would require some testing.

I agreed to the testing and five days later I returned to see Dr. Casey. She explained that I sustained quite a lot of kidney function loss and that I probably had Polycystic Kidney Disease (PKD). It could not be determined with certainly, but that I met the criteria for PKD more closely than any other kidney disease.

Dr. Casey explained that PKD is an inherited disease that causes cysts to form in the kidneys, liver, pancreas, and other organs. These cysts are filled with fluid and are formed from normal kidney structures called tubules. Approximately 10-15 percent of PKD patients may have swelling in the walls of blood vessels in the brain called aneurysms. Aneurysms in the brain are my greatest fear.

The growth of the cysts become so numerous that they literally crowd the surrounding kidney tissue by causing pressure, which in turn decreases kidney function. Patients with kidney disease can live normal lives until they have lost 90-95 percent of kidney function. Officially, PKD does not usually occur until after 40 years of age. However, in my situation and that of my relatives, the onset was at approximately 30 to 35 years of age.

There are two types of PKD, autosomal dominant PKD where almost half of the effected patients develop chronic kidney failure between 40 to 60 years of age; and autosomal recessive PKD which causes kidney failure in early childhood.

There are more persons with PKD than the combined numbers of those with cystic fibrosis, muscular dystrophy, hemophilia, Down's syndrome and sickle cell anemia! *See Appendix (A) for more detailed information.*

CHAPTER FIVE

RELOCATION TO FLORIDA

> *"Illness is not something a person has.*
> *It's another way of being. "*
>
> -Jonathan Miller,
> The Body in Question

I sat numbly listening to what Dr. Casey was saying. I wanted to cry. To me my death seemed imminent because three of my four relatives who had kidney disease were already deceased. Given my family history, I always knew that kidney disease was a very real possibility for me. My lack of surprise at my health circumstance did not make hearing it any easier. The only question I had was, "What are my options?"

I felt a great sense of loss. Douglas and I were trying for a year to have a child. He even endured the reversal of a vasectomy so we could procreate. Having a child now seemed a mute point because it would put too much of a strain on my already impaired kidneys. If I did conceive, the worst case scenario was that I could sustain a massive stroke and die, or even worse. I could sustain a massive stroke and live, not being able to care for myself or my child.

My only consolation was the fact that I would not be passing on my disease. My life as I saw it was over. I was robbed of the chance of having what I wanted the most, a son. My only hope now was adoption. Because of my health problem, coupled with the fact that Douglas was a great deal older than myself, we believed we would be considered poor risks by any adoption agency. I also knew that at some point I would have to face dialysis and eventually transplantation.

My self image was greatly affected because I felt people would now see me as physically impaired. Apart from the usual childhood diseases and having my appendix removed at age 17, I led an otherwise healthy existence.

I wondered if it was apparent to anyone looking at me that I had a health problem. I also began to over excel at everything I did to compensate for my disease, which I initially saw as a shortcoming. Since normality has always been very important to me, I continually pushed myself to participate in all my usual activities to perpetuate the illusion that I was a "normal person."

I felt that I had nothing to look forward to. I needed a goal. I had not completed my education after I was married because we moved frequently. Here was an area on which I could focus.

Douglas lost his job and we began having financial difficulties. Five months later, we were forced to move to another state where Douglas was able to secure employment. Douglas was a Computer Systems Analyst, therefore telephone interviews were a part of the normal process. After several telephone interviews, we were presented with three possibilities of employment in Michigan, Florida and Connecticut.

We began the exhaustive process of packing and the usual difficult decisions as to what treasures to keep or discard. Meanwhile, I received and perused the tapes and other materials which, I requested from the Chamber of Commerce offices in the cities of each state for which Douglas had interviewed.

With my research completed, I was prepared for our impending move. Two weeks before our departure, we were told that we were being sent to Florida. I experienced a degree of panic because I knew nothing about the city we were going to. The city was not the one originally mentioned. I rushed out and bought a map of the state of Florida and looked for the city's location. I have to confess that I was not too thrilled with the prospect because I had my heart set on relocating to Connecticut. With very little enthusiasm and with no small measure of trepidation, I continued preparing for our move. Finally the day arrived, and with all our belongings in a twenty-four foot truck and with my Mazda RX-7 in tow, we left Colorado and my heart.

The trip took us three days, during which time our main challenge was keeping our pair of Miniature Dobermans, Red Sonja and Kalidor, fed, watered and entertained. To accomplish this we stopped every four hours to stretch our legs and walk the dogs.

We arrived in Florida when the state was experiencing one of the hottest summers ever recorded and the humidity was close to one hundred percent. Having just left Colorado with its moderate temperatures and almost zero percent humidity all year round, I thought I would surely die of heat prostration.

I resigned myself to the fact that Florida would be my home for several years, and began the task of settling in and acquainting myself with my surroundings.

Three days later, I began experiencing lightheadedness and felt very sleepy most of the time. It took me forever to unpack because I was forced to sleep a great portion of the day. Hoping that I had not contracted some dreaded exotic disease, I went to see my new physician.

As is customary on a first appointment, I gave the internist my medical history. When I was through speaking he said, "No one is going to care that you have kidney disease." Then he asked, "What do you expect me to do for you?" I said that I required monthly monitoring. Tests needed to be ordered to establish a baseline, and each month the tests were to be repeated for comparison.

It was the only way I could measure the progress of my disease and track the rate at which I was losing kidney function. I further stated that these tests required a physician's request.

He reluctantly agreed to order my baseline tests and he promised a telephone call from his office with the test results would be forthcoming. Several weeks went by without a word, and finally, I telephoned and requested the test results. The internist explained that my lightheadedness was a result of adjusting to being at sea level after having moved to Florida from the Mile High City, Denver, Colorado.

For the following three months, we observed the same routine of me calling to have my tests ordered, and calling again for the results. I decided that I had made a mistake in selecting my primary care physician and resolved to find another physician in whom I had more confidence.

CHAPTER SIX

CONSULTATION WITH
MY TRANSPLANT SURGEON

> *"....we have a tendency to obscure the forest*
> *of simple joys with the trees of problems."*
>
> -Christiane Collange

During our first two years in Florida I did not lose any kidney function. Unfortunately, my relationship with Douglas, which had been deteriorating for several years, deteriorated even further, ending my nine-year marriage. Douglas subsequently relocated to another state. This circumstance was in no way related to my health problem. I was not thoroughly unlucky, however, because I managed to secure employment as a Medical Secretary with one of the best medical facilities where the salary was competitive and the benefits were outstanding.

I took one of the physicians I worked for into my confidence. I explained my health situation, then asked him, "If you needed to see a nephrologist, who would you see?" Two days later he got back to me with the name of a nephrologist several of his colleagues had recommended. The nephrologist was Dr. Ivan Thornton.

On my first visit with Dr. Thornton, I felt as though we had an instant rapport. He was thorough and he answered my questions to my satisfaction. Glancing at my medical history, he read aloud, "No tobacco or alcohol use, no tea or coffee." Then he looked at me and asked, "Come on, tell me the truth, you are doing the good stuff aren't you, heroine, cocaine?" His unique sense of humor made it clear to me then that we were going to get along.

Dr. Thornton did ask why I switched physicians, so I related my unfortunate experience with the first nephrologist I had seen at another medical facility.

He responded by saying, "Patients should not change their physicians arbitrarily or on a whim, but, if necessary to obtain the best medical care, they should not hesitate to make a change. It is every patient's right and that right should not be denied." I did not have any qualms then about placing my life in his very capable hands.

As my disease progressed, I kept in touch with my brother, Michael, who kept me apprised about what to expect, since his disease was much further advanced than mine. Also, my sister, Joanne, had returned to Trinidad to take care of Michael who was now on hemodialysis.

The day I was supposed to begin my new job, I received a telephone call from Joanne advising me that Michael had died. After a lengthy conversation punctuated by crying, I telephoned my supervisor to advise her that I would not be at work that day. She was very empathetic.

I could only imagine what my father must be feeling. He had lost his wife and now a son. "A man is not supposed to outlive his children," he said. In the midst of his grief, I am sure the possibility of losing me as well had not escaped him.

Over the following months, there were two major signs that my disease was progressing. The first sign was a lack of energy. To counteract this, Dr. Thornton decided to initiate Epogen® injections. Epogen® (erythropoietin) is a growth hormone which is normally produced by the kidneys. Erythropoietin stimulates the bone marrow to produce red blood cells. Dialysis patients do not produce enough erythropoietin, consequently they become anemic. Erythropoietin can be injected subcutaneously or directly into the tubing during dialysis treatments.

These injections were extremely painful and produced a significant amount of bruising. I learned that the injections would be significantly less painful if the Epogen® was allowed to achieve room temperature and administered in the subcutaneous tissue of the abdomen. On the day of my next Epogen® injection I requested that the injection be given in my abdomen. It seemed such an unnatural area for injections that it made me queasy.

Once the injection was over, I was shaken but was pleasantly surprised that I had experienced minimal discomfort. From that time forward, I always held my vial of Epogen® in my hands to warm it before it was administered, and I continued the injections in my abdominal area.

The second indication that my disease was progressing was the elevation of my BUN and Creatinine levels. When my creatinine achieved a level of 6 mg/dL (normal 0-1 mg/dL), Dr. Thornton suggested a consultation with a transplant surgeon. Once again I did my research and discovered that the surgeon was highly recommended and had a very high kidney transplant success rate. I was comfortable with this information and called for an appointment.

I was very excited when I went to my initial consultation with Dr. Mark Taber. He explained the criteria for being placed on the kidney transplant waiting list, which include: health condition, age, and whether or not I had any other health problems which would preclude transplantation as a viable option.

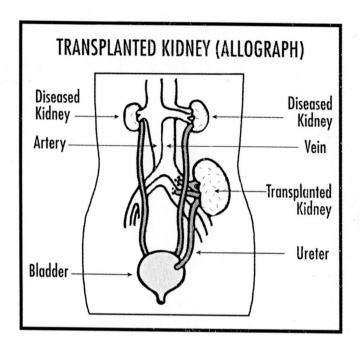

TRANSPLANTED KIDNEY (ALLOGRAPH)

Diseased Kidney

Artery

Bladder

Diseased Kidney

Vein

Transplanted Kidney

Ureter

Dr. Taber further explained that a kidney transplant is a procedure that places a healthy kidney from another person into my body. The surgeon places the kidney in my body between my upper thigh and abdomen. The artery and vein from the new kidney are attached to my artery and vein. My blood flows through the transplanted kidney and makes urine. The new kidney may start working right away or take up to a few weeks or months to work. My native kidneys are not removed unless they become infected, or enlarged by disease and cause discomfort, or hypertension.

I may receive a kidney from a family member (living-related donor) or a kidney from someone who has recently died (cadaver donor). The donor's blood and tissue has to match mine closely. The average waiting period for a cadaver kidney while on the kidney transplant list is 6-12 months.

The greater the blood compatibility shared by a donor and the recipient, the greater the chance of a successful transplant. An ABO blood test is the first test done to determine compatibility. People are identified as blood type A, B, AB, or O. Type O is the most common, followed by type A. Only a small percentage of the population has type B or type AB. The following table shows to whom a person can give a kidney, or from whom a person can receive a kidney, based on blood type.

BLOOD TYPE	CAN RECEIVE FROM TYPE	CAN DONATE TO TYPE
O	O	O, A, B, AB
A	A, O	A, AB
B	B, O	B, AB
AB	O, A, B, AB	AB

On average, the surgery usually takes approximately two to three hours. The average hospital stay is one week and recuperating time would depend solely on my body's resiliency. The transplanted kidney will work in the same way as my native kidneys used to. Gender, and age of my donor kidney does not matter. Age can play an indirect role because HLA antigens do vary by race.

I could resume a normal diet and there will be no further need for dialysis. On the other hand, a transplant is major surgery. My transplanted kidney may not last a lifetime and I may require another transplant. I may suffer a rejection episode and will be taking various medications for the rest of my life.

My transplant team will consist of my doctors, nurses, social workers, pharmacists, dietitians, and transplant coordinator. My transplant physician will see me every day while in the hospital. The transplant surgeon will actually be transplanting my new kidney into my body. My transplant coordinator, a registered nurse, will be coordinating all facets of my transplant, from obtaining a donor kidney, overseeing pre-transplant tests, education, exercise program and follow-up care post transplantation.

The social worker will be responsible for answering any questions that I have regarding Medicare, disability insurance, other sources of financial assistance, providing information on support groups and counseling. My dietitian will provide nutritional information and the pharmacist will provide vital information about my medications. I may need various other health professionals as needed, but the most important member of my team will be myself. In other words, I have to educate myself, keep a positive mental attitude, after all I am my own best friend and closest ally. I am my own best motivator.

I reviewed, at length, the list of medications I would be taking. The literature that I was given stressed the importance of taking the medications exactly as directed and never missing a dose. This could result in a rejection episode and ultimately the loss of my transplanted kidney. I would also be required to measure my urine output, measure intake, take my temperature every day, weigh each morning, and above all, I must call the Transplant Center if I experience any of the following: headache, chills, fever, weight gain over two pounds, nausea, vomiting and/or diarrhea.

The symptoms which accompany a rejection episode include: decrease in urine output, water retention, pain or soreness over the kidney, fever, swelling of feet and ankles, weight gain, increase in blood pressure and a general feeling of being ill. Some additional symptoms could be pain or burning during urination, blood or odor in the urine, coughing, shortness of breath, nausea, vomiting, headache, fatigue, weakness and irritability. I was advised to call my transplant team immediately if I experienced any of the above listed symptoms.

Experiencing a rejection episode does not necessarily mean that I am losing the transplanted kidney. I could have an infection which is easily contracted because of my immunosuppression.

Several medications are used to treat a rejection episode: Solu-Medrol®, Prednisone®, OKT3®, Prograf® or Rapamune® which are administered intravenously. Change in dosage of immunosuppressive medicines and dialysis may also be required until rejection subsides and kidney function increases.

Possible side effects of immunosuppressant medications include: increase or loss of appetite, weakness, dizziness, itching, fuller face, weight gain, excessive hair growth and weakened immune system.

Of special note, was our discussion on blood pressure and the need to check it daily. Normal blood pressure ranges between 110/70 and 140/90 mm/Hg. The top number is called the systolic blood pressure, which is the force at which the heart muscle contracts and blood is pumped out of the heart chambers. The bottom number is called the diastolic blood pressure, which measures the force of the heart muscle as it expands and fills with blood. By monitoring my blood pressure at home I can determine whether my blood pressure is under control. High blood pressure reflects changes in kidney function, side effects of the medications, or too much sodium in my diet.

Dr. Taber continued by adding that transplantation is not a cure. The average life span of a transplanted kidney is ten years. Some patients have only one transplant which lasts their entire life, and other less fortunate patients require several transplants during their lifetime. I also discovered that the main factors affecting a donor's ability to surviving transplantation are age and medical condition.

There is no limit on the amount of transplants a patient could receive. The only potentially limiting factor could be a high Patient Reactive Antibody (PRA) level, making the patient highly sensitized (after a previous transplant[s]) and very difficult to match.

Dr. Taber then described the surgical process. He said that an incision approximately 8-10 inches long would be made above the groin area on the right or the left side of the lower abdomen.

Transplantation of the new kidney would be accomplished by attaching the artery and vein of the new kidney to my artery and vein, and the kidney's ureter. After surgery, I would have a central venous line placed just above or below my collarbone for the purpose of monitoring my central venous pressure (CVP). It is also useful in obtaining blood samples and checking fluid levels. This central line would be left in place for 3-14 days.

I would also have a Foley catheter in place for the voiding of urine. I would also be expected to breathe deeply and cough to avoid contracting pneumonia. If I experience pain while coughing, I was advised to place a pillow against my abdominal area and apply light pressure to minimize the pain.

Once the consultation was over, the transplant coordinator began making arrangements for my pre-transplant workup, which would determine my eligibility for placement on the kidney transplant waiting list. Dr. Taber needed to be sure that I did not have an underlying health problem which would require correction prior to transplantation.

A pre-transplant workup includes: blood counts, chemistry profiles, and other specific tests to determine clotting ability, presence or absence of viral and bacterial infection, and kidney and bladder function.

CHAPTER SEVEN

PRE-TRANSPLANT WORKUP

> *"Difficult times have helped me to understand better than before
> how infinitely rich and beautiful life is in every way and that
> so many things that one goes worrying about are of no
> importance whatsoever."*
>
> **-Isak Dinesen**

As end-stage renal failure progresses, there are not many activities that dialysis or kidney patients are able to participate in due to lack of energy. However, many patients rehabilitate and regain an acceptable level of energy once Epogen® injections are initiated. There are many activities including assembling jigsaw puzzles, reading and making hand-crafted items, which usually do not require much in the way of energy and participating in such activities gives patients an element of control in an otherwise uncontrollable situation.

With the advent of the Easter season, Katy Tatum, a friend and co-worker, taught Sarah Walker, another dear friend and co-worker, and myself, how to make easter bunny baskets which we sold and actually made a small profit on. Such was our enjoyment of creating the baskets that we had a difficult time parting with them. At some point in the process, the bunnies each took on a personality of their own. We felt as though we were selling our children. Once we had each sold our first basket and had the money in our hands, it became easier to part with the others. Sarah, Katy and I called ourselves Her's, Her's, & Her's. I thought I was a very clever person for coming up with the name.

We all liked the name because it meant we were equal partners and no one person received top billing. This also meant that we sank or swam together. Once the Easter season was over, we decided to have a craft show in November dedicated entirely to Christmas items. We began by recruiting other crafters because we three alone could not produce enough items for an entire show.

To do this, we placed advertisements in several local newspapers and on television's Channel 4. Once we had recruited a sufficient number of crafters we began interviewing, which included a perusal of the crafter's wares. At the end of the process, we had recruited twenty-two crafters to participate in our show. Katy, Sarah and I were all experiencing trials of one kind or another, so this show was an excellent way to occupy our time and minds, and kept us from focusing on our respective challenges.

In the midst of all our preparations for the show, Sarah flexed her time at work so she could be available to take me to St. Michael's hospital for my pre-transplant workup. I was pre-admitted to the hospital several days before, so it was just a matter of signing in and waiting to be taken to my assigned room.

On our way to the hospital, we crossed the wrong bridge, which led us away from downtown and St. Michael's Hospital. We were then forced to take a circuitous route to the hospital and arrived fifteen minutes late. This was typical for Sarah and myself, because we frequently got lost on our jaunts together. Sarah had tears in her eyes as she hugged me goodbye and said, "I hate the fact that you have to go through this. I don't want to leave you here." I asked her not to cry, I needed to keep my spirits high, besides I have a strict philosophy, that no one cries alone in my presence.

The following 48 hours were grueling. The VCU (voiding cystourethrogram) was my least favorite of all the tests. I was catheterized and my bladder was filled with dye. While standing up, I was then required to urinate into a special collecting apparatus placed snugly between the top of my thighs, as a technician took x-rays of the passage of the dye through my ureters and bladder. The purpose of this test was to determine whether or not I was experiencing reflux of urine in my ureters and whether or not my bladder was emptying completely.

Because I have what is termed a bashful bladder, I was advised by a nurse to practice urinating while standing up in the shower. This was a distasteful prospect, but it worked.

Forty-eight hours later, the testing was completed and I was ready to go home. Sarah came to pick me up and said very little. I could tell by the look on her face that I looked terrible. I was also very hungry and had a yen for a grilled chicken sandwich, French fries and a lemonade. A hospital stay always gives me an appreciation for fast food.

Upon arriving at my apartment, Sarah asked if there was anything else she could do for me. Being the comedian I like to think I am, I said, "It seems to me that every time I am admitted to a hospital to have awful things done to me, you are always the one to take me there. No thank you! I believe you've done enough!" We both laughed and again I thought how good life was. Several days later, I received a letter formally advising me of the favorable results of my pre-transplant workup and that I had been placed on the kidney transplant waiting list.

The following steps in the process were appointments with a nephrologist, a social worker, and a transplant coordinator who would be assigning me a pocket pager. I was strongly urged to wear my pocket pager at all times, and check the batteries periodically.

I was also advised to always leave a number where the Transplant Center could contact me, especially if I planned to travel. The distance traveled should not exceed four hours from home, and I had fifteen minutes in which to respond to a page and eight hours to wait for the results of the blood tests. I must not eat or drink anything from the time of the first phone call. Once I officially accept the offer of a kidney, I must proceed to the hospital immediately, because although the donor kidney is stored in [University of Wisconsin (UW)] solution to keep it suitable for transplantation, there is a time limit.

Both Dr. Thornton and myself had hoped that I would be transplanted before the initiation of dialysis, but it was not to be. I began feeling very tired and my walking became labored. I felt a deep seated exhaustion which seemed to penetrate my bones. At first I thought I was suffering from dehydration or low blood pressure, since these produce similar symptoms.

During the onset of these new symptoms, I often spent weekends at a lake with friends. I was probably perceived as a bore because I spent most of the time sitting quietly and reading. I could not participate in the activities because I lacked the energy to do so. Just walking back and fourth from the water's edge produced a deep aching in my legs, buttocks and back. Brushing my teeth and chewing food became challenges. I needed to rest every few strokes while brushing my teeth and was forced to pause while chewing food to alleviate the aching in my jaws.

Chewing became so labored that I began having steamed vegetables, oatmeal, mashed potatoes, or soup for every meal. The thought of eating a salad filled me with dread. It was not worth the effort, pain, or length of time it would take me to consume an entire salad. Washing and blow drying my hair, and applying makeup also required a tremendous amount of effort and on occasion, took me, approximately two hours to complete the process. Consequently, to be on time for my appointments, I had to have an early start. A few weeks later, I began experiencing nausea, vomiting and lightheadedness.

I telephoned Dr. Thornton and related my list of symptoms. He said that he had just received my latest laboratory results and my creatinine was now 8.0 mg/dL (normal 0-1.0 mg/dL) and my BUN was 80 mg/dL (normal 6-19 mg/dL). He then said that it was time to initiate dialysis. I was instructed to go to the ER (emergency room) at St. Ignatius Hospital. He would phone ahead so I would be expected. He also ordered the placement of the first in a long line of Quinton® catheters (direct accesses for dialysis). My heart sank and I thought how awful life was.

Within minutes of my arrival at St. Ignatius hospital, a whirlwind of activity began around me. An IV was placed, blood was drawn and a catheterized urine specimen was obtained. A physician then entered the room and said, "You don't look as though you have anything wrong." To which I responded, "My laboratory results say otherwise." I was then told that I was a special patient. I could not help but be grateful to be a "special patient," I hated to think how they would treat a VIP. When in doubt, go for the joke I always say. It is always better to laugh than cry.

Transplant patients lead a very precarious life. Its as though we are walking on a sidewalk strewn with banana peels. One moment you are going merrily along, the next, you slip and down you go. For this reason I believe that a life threatening disease is the most humbling of experiences. During times of great trial or stress, I learned that I had to hang on to my sense of humor. Without a sense of humor I would not have survived what was to follow in the next three years.

The physician re-entered the room with the results of my tests which were run on a STAT basis. He could not believe that I drove myself to the ER or could walk with a creatinine which had increased to 9 mg/dL. If he had not seen the laboratory results himself, he would not have believed it. A huge drawback with PKD is that I never looked as though I had anything wrong, consequently I never got any sympathy. Not that sympathy was what I wanted or needed.

It is very difficult for your friends and co-workers to understand and accept that although you look terrific, you feel dreadful. Each time someone said that I did not look as though I had a health problem, I think back to my mother's funeral. She too did not look as though she had a health problem while lying lifeless in her casket.

During this chain of events, I had to make an extra effort to maintain a positive attitude. I felt as though my body was literally falling apart and there was nothing I could do to control it. I felt helpless. All I could do was pray and trust that my Heavenly Father would see me through and I would survive.

There were moments, however, when even prayer sometimes gave little comfort. I needed something more tangible, such as a hug or a sympathetic ear. In this respect, I was very fortunate because I had a wide circle of friends which I hope the good Lord will bless immeasurably for providing me with an incredible support system and ultimately my sanity saver. I also had two mentors, both kidney transplant patients themselves who were only a phone call away.

CHAPTER EIGHT

HEMODIALYSIS

*"When one door of happin ess closes, another opens;
but often we look so long at the closed door that we do not
see the one which has been opened for us."*
-Helen Keller

    The placement of my first Quinton® catheter was uneventful and produced a minor amount of discomfort. This was due to the fact that I was lightly sedated. The catheter was placed in my right internal jugular vein, as a temporary access for dialysis. The catheter is a thin tube which is divided into two parts. One side is used to draw blood to the dialyzer. The other side is used to return the dialyzed blood back to me.

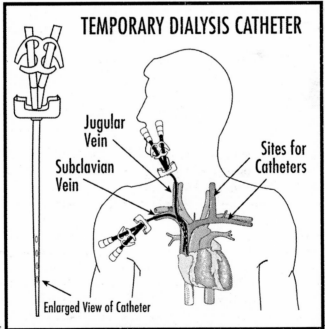

TEMPORARY DIALYSIS CATHETER

Jugular Vein

Subclavian Vein

Sites for Catheters

Enlarged View of Catheter

    This [..] the right side of my neck. You can always tell Lidocaine® because of its distinctive sting. Then an incision was made and the catheter inserted. I felt twinges as though the catheter was catching on its way down to its resting place. Next, an x-ray was taken to check for proper placement of the catheter. I was then admitted to the hospital and taken to my room. Later than night when the effects of the Lidocaine® had worn off, I experienced a considerable amount of pain.

A permanent dialysis catheter is similar to a temporary dialysis catheter in appearance, and because of the following special features, it can be left in place longer.

* It is made of a soft silicone material.
* A Dacron® cuff is tunneled under the skin to provide a germ barrier and an anchor to hold it in place.

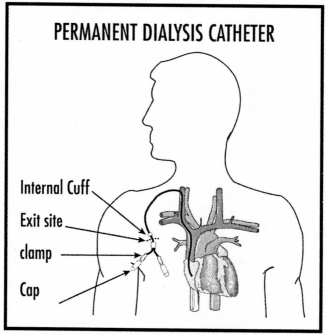

PERMANENT DIALYSIS CATHETER

Internal Cuff
Exit site
clamp
Cap

In the midst of my pain, a female patient barged into my room and in a very loud voice she asked, "What are you in for?" I replied, "Dialysis." The patient then asked again in a very loud voice, "What is dialysis?" Before I could respond, two nurses entered my room and promptly escorted the patient back to her room across the hall.

The following morning at 7:30 a.m., the dialysis nurses Lisa and Madeline came to take me to dialysis. As they attempted to wheel me out of my room, bed and all, the doorway was blocked by the same female patient who visited me the previous day. She was closely followed by two nurses who were struggling to remove her from the doorway. She hung onto my bed, yelling, "Here," as she handed me her medications.

I extended my hand, took the medications, said, "Thank you," and promptly handed them to one of the nurses in attendance. The nurses managed to shake her hold on my bed and took her back to her room. That just served to reinforce the fact that you never know what to expect in life.

Finally, we arrived at the Dialysis Department and the nurses proceeded to hook me up for my first dialysis treatment. The treatment only lasted for two hours, but to me, it felt as though it was six. In an attempt to take my mind off the discomfort and assuage my anxiety, the nurse proceeded to explain the hemodialysis process.

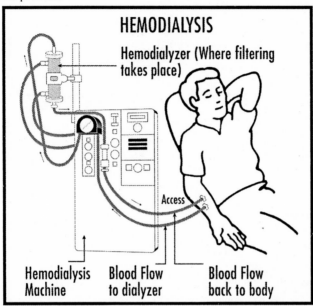

She began by saying that healthy kidneys clean the blood by filtering out extra water, salt, fluids and wastes. The kidneys also control blood pressure and helps the body maintain proper balance of potassium, sodium and chloride. The kidneys also produce hormones that maintain strong bones and healthy blood. Patients with end-stage renal disease (ESRD) are hypertensive, their bodies retain water, there is a build-up of harmful wastes, and their bone marrow no longer produces red blood cells without the aid of erythropoietin.

The hemodialysis machine takes the place of the kidneys, in that, it acts as a filtration unit for certain waste products. It accomplishes this by using a special filter to clean the blood. The dialysis machine is divided in two parts. They are separated by a very thin sheet of plastic with millions of tiny holes. Red blood cells are too large to pass through these holes. The dialyzer actually filters the wastes and excess water, as these particles are smaller and fit through the holes in the filter. The cleaned blood (including red blood cells) then flows through another set of tubes and back into the body.

This process is accomplished through the use of an access to the bloodstream called a fistula or graft. In my case, this took the form of a segment of Gortex® attached to an artery and a vein which was embedded in my left lower arm.

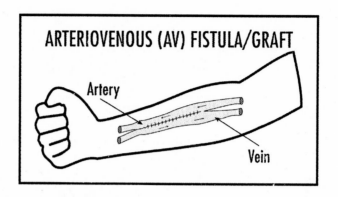

ARTERIOVENOUS (AV) FISTULA/GRAFT

Artery

Vein

Hemodialysis can be done at home or at a center with trained technicians and nurses. Hemodialysis is usually performed three times a week for two to four hours each treatment. During treatment sudden changes of fluid balance can cause side effects such as muscle cramps, hypotension (drop in blood pressure), a general feeling of weakness, dizziness, nausea, chest pain or "squeezing" pressure on my chest, sudden chills or heavy sweating and severe or unusual pain.

If I experience any of these problems, I should be certain to tell my dialysis care team. The care team can often fix these problems in one of two ways: slowing down the rate at which sodium and water are taken out of my body during dialysis or changing the type of cleansing bath used in the dialysis machine. These symptoms can also be minimized by following a few simple rules: eating a balanced diet, limiting fluid intake, limiting potassium intake, avoiding salt, and limiting foods such as, dairy products, nuts, dried beans, and soft drinks. During treatment, the dialysis care team will check my weight, blood pressure, pulse and temperature. A sample of my blood is also taken at regular times for testing.

Dialysis is not a cure, at best, it is maintenance. It does not stop the progression of PKD. A diet and exercise regimen is extremely important to maintain a certain level of energy. Many older patients opt to stay on dialysis rather than try a transplant. Some do not want to take all the medications involved, especially the immunosuppressants.

I was told that I could live a long healthy life on dialysis. This thought brought me no end of comfort. Another comforting thought was that end-stage renal disease (ESRD) patients are living longer than ever and although problems develop as ESRD progresses, doctors have new and better ways of preventing or treating them.

I could opt for In-center Hemodialysis where treatments are scheduled by the center, and I would have trained professionals with me at all times, I would get to know the other patients, and I would gain a sense of independence and control over my treatments. Or I could choose Home Hemodialysis. I would need training, I could do it at the hours I choose, I do not have to travel to a center, helping with treatments may be stressful to my family, and I need space for storing the machine and supplies at home.

Whichever type my doctor and I decided to try, I would still have to be stuck with needles every time I have to dialyze. I hated being stuck with those big needles because I found the procedure to be very painful. Also, during treatments, too much water, sodium or potassium would be removed from my blood stream too rapidly, causing uncomfortable symptoms. Once the treatment was completed and the needles were removed, I disliked having to sit for twenty minutes applying direct pressure to the area waiting for the bleeding to stop. I also disliked the fact that I felt so weak after each treatment, that I was only capable of eating and sleeping.

Dialysis treatments must be permanent because waste products will build up in my blood between treatments, dialysis has to be done every few days. I will need dialysis for the rest of my life. The only way I can stop dialysis is to have a successful kidney transplant.

Once I begin hemodialysis, I will be at high risk for bone disease. For this reason, all dialysis patients have to be placed on a low-phosphorus diet, which unfortunately, also happens to be low in calcium. Because of this, dialysis patients usually do not get enough calcium to maintain healthy bones. Also, the kidneys of dialysis patients do not make enough calcitriol, the "active" form of Vitamin D, which helps the body absorb and use calcium. Calcium supplements are therefore necessary

Calcium is the basic "bone builder." Calcitriol is the "guide," helping to send calcium to the bones and stopping it from leaving the body as waste. Calcitriol also helps feed the bone cells so they grow correctly. Some phosphorus too, is also required for the bones. However, too much phosphorus is not good; it can hurt the bones. The kidneys prevent bone disease by acting as controllers. They make Vitamin D active so it can help send calcium to the bones.

When there is too much phosphorus, the kidneys send some of this extra phosphorus into the urine. So, since the kidneys can no longer control calcium and phosphorus, they therefore, have to be controlled through diet.

This will prevent the muscles and bones becoming weak and painful, and lower the danger of bones breaking. Should I be troubled with pain in my bones or joints, itchy skin or weak muscles, and trouble holding my arms up, I was told to report these problems immediately to my doctor or nurse. I was also told that severe itching over my entire body was a sure sign that my phosphorous level was too high. All foods have phosphorus in them.

If my phosphorus level becomes too high, it can make the calcium in my blood too low. It is therefore most important that most of the phosphorus I consume become part of the waste products which are removed from my blood stream during the dialysis process. For this purpose, phosphorus binders such as Tums® and PhosLo® are prescribed and usually taken with meals. Foods rich in phosphorus should be avoided or consumed in limited quantities. *See Appendix (B) for a list of phosphorus-rich foods.*

CHAPTER NINE

ANXIETY ATTACKS AND THERAPY

> *"If you really want to be happy, nobody can stop you."*
> **-Sister Mary Tricky**

While I was engaged in adjusting to my new way of life, diet, and medications, Sarah and Katy were occupied with sending contracts to our crafters for their signature. There was still much to do though, such as, apply for a tax ID number, open a bank account in our company's name and decide where to have our show. Sarah volunteered her home.

While Sarah and Katy occupied what little spare time they had with the preparations for the craft show, I was running the gambit of all typical problems which could occur during dialysis treatment, these were: nausea, vomiting, diarrhea, cramps in my legs, lightheadedness and generally feeling very cold. It took a few sessions before both the nurses and myself were familiar with my needs relative to dialysis. By this I mean, what was my dry weight? How much water needed to be removed? How much Epogen® I would require and how often, and appropriate changes in diet.

Because I always felt very cold after hemodialysis treatments, I could hardly wait to go out into the sunlight so I could feel its warmth on my face. Once I was strong enough to drive myself to and from treatments, it became my habit to sit in my sun-heated car with the windows rolled up, and soak in the heat.

I could feel my body relaxing and my joints stop aching as the heat slowly seeped into my body. This after-dialysis ritual became one of my most enjoyable self fulfilling pleasures.

Once I arrived home, I went to the refrigerator for something to eat. I was always ravenous after treatments. After eating, I usually spent the rest of the day in bed sleeping, because I lacked the energy to do anything else. I would awaken feeling refreshed after approximately five to six hours of sleep.

About 9 p.m., the night after one of my hemodialysis treatments, Sarah visited me and while she was speaking I suddenly sat bolt upright and looked around the room while clutching my chest. I felt very cold and tingly, my heart beat and breathing became erratic and I felt as though all the blood had been drained from my body. As I looked around the room, there seemed to be an absence of color. I was suddenly filled with fear and felt as though I was 200 percent certain I was dying. Sarah, wide-eyed, asked what was wrong.

She said that I sat up and all the color drained from my face and I seemed to stare at the wall. I described to her how I felt and what I saw, and that I thought that I was dying. To which Sarah asked, "What, right now!" I said, "Yes." Sarah went in search of a nurse who checked my vital signs and found them to be indeed elevated. I was given 2.5 mg of Xanax® and a few minutes later I felt better.

This strange occurrence I realized later took place only on dialysis days and usually around 9 p.m. I would not be able to sit, stand, or lie down for fear of dying. I felt as though I needed to speak to someone or look someone in the eyes to keep me grounded and alive. During one of these episodes, I looked at myself in the mirror and said, "You are fine, apart from your kidney failure, the doctors could not find anything else wrong with you. Your heart and lungs are fine and you are receiving excellent medical care. There is no earthly reason for you to believe you're dying." Dr. Thornton called these strange occurrences anxiety attacks.

To me the attacks seemed to be illogical. I was doing very well, all things considered. Why did I have this unfounded fear and not be able to control it no matter what I did? Prayer did not seem to have any effect. I needed help. I could not battle this alone. I asked Dr. Thornton for a referral to a therapist.

On my first visit with the therapist, we did nothing but talk. He asked me why I thought I needed to see him. I explained that I wanted to know what was at the root of my anxiety attacks and what my options were for controlling them without the use of medication. I began at the beginning, and as I talked the therapist took notes. After the first page of handwritten notes he looked up at me and said, "Enough," but I continued to speak.

When I finally stopped speaking, he looked up at me and said, "I am not surprised that you are having some problems. I cannot believe how much you've been through in the last two years." He asked me several more questions and after listening carefully to my answers he said, "I think that you are one of the most sane people I have ever met. I sense that you are a person who has always been able to cope with whatever life has thrown your way. Now, you are dealing with too many major issues at the same time and you are overwhelmed. You need a little help to get you through this rough time. You probably just need someone to talk to. Do you have a good support system in place?" I said that I did, but I felt the need to speak to a health care professional to assure myself of my mental stability.

The day after my appointment with the therapist, I began biofeedback, relaxation techniques and meditation. At some of my appointments, I merely talked about the current and past events of my life. It felt wonderful to unload my problems, it was positively liberating. After about a month, I felt much better and back in control and discontinued the sessions. It was a relief to know that I was only over stressed and not completely off my trolley. Of course my friends might disagree. I found myself fighting psychological, physical, and emotional battles, sometimes all at the same time. The stakes were high. What else did I possess that was worth more than my life. I felt a certain sense of urgency to come up with a game plan to keep my psyche together, and maintain a positive outlook.

I became aware of the amount of negativity surrounding me. I frequently found myself angry at any injustice I saw on the news or crying over certain television commercials. Therefore, I embarked on a campaign to replace all the negativity in my own private world with positive thoughts and activities. The first step was making a list of positive affirmations, especially geared to my needs. I began each morning by reciting these affirmations aloud before I got out of bed. I also constantly bombarded myself with uplifting music and books.

I stopped watching the news and only viewed uplifting movies on television. Each time I had a negative thought, I would say, "Cancel, cancel," to myself and replace the negative thought with a positive one. I also made a tremendous effort to avoid getting upset, angry or feeling self-pity. I pushed myself everyday to get out of bed, apply my make-up and get dressed. I found that when I looked good I felt good, and when I felt good I did better mentally, physically and emotionally. Volunteering a few hours a week for my local Kidney Foundation was of great benefit, because it lifted my spirits and kept me strong. Because of this strength, I never used my health as an excuse for anything.

I continued my treatments at the Dialysis Clinic, 7 a.m., every Tuesday, Thursday, and Saturday for two hours each session. As my disease progressed, the duration of my treatments grew in proportion from two, to three, then three and a half hours. To get through these treatments, I took 2.5 mg of Xanax® and 325 mg of Percocet® half an hour before each treatment, so I could sleep through the entire process.

On my following visit with Dr. Thornton, he advised me that my Quinton® catheter was a temporary means of accomplishing my dialysis and could only be used for a maximum period of six weeks due to risk of infection. It was time to schedule the placement of a permanent access for my hemodilysis.

On one occasion during a hemodialysis treatment I felt a tickle on my neck and down my chest. I reached up to scratch and my hand came in contact with something moist. I looked at my fingertips and found them covered in blood. I then looked down at my chest and realized that there was a trickle of blood running from the point of insertion of the Quinton® catheter in the right side of my neck, and down to my cleavage. I called for help.

The nurse came over and told me that it was my fault that I was bleeding. "You should not be scratching your neck," she said. In actuality, the dialysis machine was running at a higher rate than I could tolerate. I improved when the machine was run at a slower rate and I tolerated dialysis much better. Because of the slower rate, however, my treatments had to be extended for a longer period of time, so I would be adequately dialyzed.

The next time I saw Dr. Thornton, he suggested proceeding with effecting a natural fistula in the area of my right wrist. This required a visit with a vascular surgeon and surgery under general anesthesia. The following day, while I was being prepped for surgery, I took a long look at my right wrist, since I knew that I would never see it in such a pristine condition again. The usual medications were administered and I was taken to the OR where my natural fistula was created by grafting an artery to a vein. I awoke to a horrendous throbbing in my right wrist.

I was told that pain would be worst in those areas because there are many more nerve ending in the extremities. Needless to say I began taking Percocet® in four hour intervals for the next few days for pain control. Every time my vital signs were checked, the fistula was checked for signs of a bruit (a sound or murmur heard in auscultation). This caused me no joy since the fistula began throbbing each time it was touched. I was given a "Hand Helper®" (device or ball you squeeze) to increase the size and strength of my vessel to achieve an adequate blood flow for dialysis. I was instructed to begin using the Hand Helper® in approximately two weeks time. I should exercise four to six times a day and each session should last for no more than five to ten minutes. *See Appendix (C) for the care of a fistula and fistula arm.*

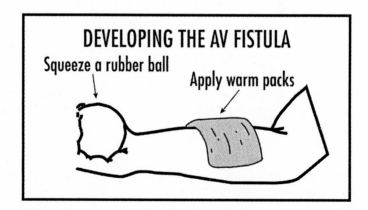

DEVELOPING THE AV FISTULA
Squeeze a rubber ball
Apply warm packs

At 2:30 a.m., the following morning, the nurse came in to check my vital signs and my fistula. She had a concerned look on her face. A physician was summoned from the ER and he confirmed the nurse's worst suspicion, no thrill and no bruit. The fistula had failed. Again I thought how awful life is. A second visit to the vascular surgeon was required. This time a straight Gortex® graft would be placed from my left wrist to my antecubital fossa (bend in the arm opposite the elbow).

Throughout the night, I had a recurring thought. If the fistula which only had a 4 percent chance of failing, had in fact failed, what would be the odds of having success with the Gortex® graft, since I had small and delicate veins. I remembered several dialysis patients telling me that failed fistulas and the creation of new ones are a fact of life for dialysis patients.

Each day brings a new challenge to the dialysis patient. Some of these challenges include: a blood pressure which is either too high or too low, abnormal laboratory values requiring constant changes in diet and medications and clotting blood accesses, just to name a few.

Dealing with these issues was a very delicate juggling act and required a huge amount of intestinal fortitude. Sometimes, patients are unable to cope and are plunged into deep depression. So great is their depression that they refuse their life-saving dialysis treatments and would rather die.

I envisioned myself with an accumulation of scars up and down both arms as the result of failed fistulas, like many of the patients at the Dialysis Center. I was fearful. I knew that if I did not have my kidney transplant before I ran out of sites for blood accesses, I would be out of options. I telephoned Joanne and asked if her offer of a kidney was still available; she said yes. The following day she began making arrangements to fly to Florida. I made an appointment for the day after Joanne's arrival for her to be Human Leukocyte Antigen (HLA) tested and crossmatched for compatibility. The HLA testing/HLA Crossmatch is performed by mixing blood of the donor and recipient to determine if the recipient can receive an organ, tissue, or blood from the donor.

I informed Dr. Thornton that I had decided not to proceed with the placement of the Gortex® graft. I was discharged from the hospital the following day. I had one week to prepare for Joanne's arrival.

On the day of Joanne's arrival, my co-worker Tracy and I, arrived at the airport just in time to see the passengers disembark from the plane, but there was no sign of Joanne. I experienced a moment of panic as the thought occurred to me that she might have missed her plane. As the passengers entered the terminal and walked toward where we were standing, I realized that Joanne was one of the first to disembark. She looked so different that I did not recognize her. Her hair was longer than I had ever seen it, almost completely gray and appeared blond in the sunlight. Joanne came over immediately and gave me a hug, calling me R2D2® pointing to the Quinton® catheter in my neck.

After Joanne uttered only a few words, Tracy said, "Yep, she's your sister." I still cannot understand what she meant, it must have been the accent. The following day, after a visit to the beauty salon, we went to the hospital where I worked to introduce Joanne to my co-workers. She was an instant hit. Everyone liked her and said that it was wonderful to have her here. It was as though they now had two of me. I did not think that Florida was ready for that contingency.

After an anxious wait of eight hours, we had the result of the HLA typing. Joanne's and my HLA typing was compatible. It was a match!!! Joanne's next step was a visit with the transplant surgeon to set a date for her pre-transplant workup which would determine her eligibility to donate a kidney.

The consultation with Dr. Taber went well. Joanne's only concerns were: would she have a normal, active life after donating a kidney, would she be able to have children, and how would the loss of one kidney affect her body.

Dr. Taber explained that she would have a normal life and be as active as she wanted, and would not experience any problems having children. He further stated that with two fully functioning kidneys a normal healthy person has 10-15 times more kidney function than is required to sustain life, and with one fully functioning kidney a person has 8-10 times more kidney function than is required. He also said that when a kidney is removed, the other increases in size to compensate for the loss of the other.

My dear friends who work with me in the laboratory adopted Joanne just as they had adopted me. They brought us gifts of food, took us shopping, to movies, and sightseeing for Joanne's benefit. They also said many prayers on our behalf. They are the best. "The Blue People," that is what Joanne called them, because they all wore blue scrubs at work. Every time I think of them, and their outpouring of love, my eyes well with tears. Each time I tried to thank them their response was always the same, "Your getting well is thanks enough for us."

Meanwhile, back at work, both my employer and myself anticipated that I would be exhausting my short-term leave, then going into long-term leave. The next order of business then was to sign the "Family Leave Act," which would protect my job and guaranteed that I would have a job (not necessarily the same job) once I recovered and was ready to return to work.

CHAPTER TEN

MY SISTER GIVES ME A KIDNEY

You find yourself refreshed by the presence of cheerful people.
Why not make an honest effort to confer that pleasure
on others? Half the battle is gained if you never allow
yourself to say anything gloomy.

-Lydia M. Child

Although I was participating in the preparations for the craft show, I still felt as though I was not able to give one hundred percent. I hoped that I was not disappointing my "partners in crime." Of course, Sarah and Katy assured me this was not the case. They felt that I had enough to occupy my thoughts and that I should be preparing for the upcoming kidney transplant.

Meanwhile, the average life-span of my Quinton® catheters was about one week. They were frequently being replaced. Both ports of the catheter were filled with concentrated 500 Heparin®, and in between dialysis treatments the Heparin® was aspirated and replaced with a fresh supply of Heparin® as a further precaution against clotting. I asked Dr. Taber, "What are the chances that my new kidney would clot?" His response was, "Only two percent of all transplanted kidneys clot, and the possibility of my transplanted kidney clotting was very remote." Each time I had to have a catheter changed, I was given Valium® to keep me calm and from having anxiety attacks. Once the Valium® had taken effect, the normal procedure for removal and replacement of the catheter would be followed.

This process is not painless. Depending on the expertise of your "torturer," you could experience minimal to severe pain. During one of these exchanges I experienced severe pain. I felt as though the guide wire had struck my heart. My heart fluttered and my breathing became erratic. I could not catch my breath and there were loud noises emanating from my heart monitor. The nurse yelled to the doctor to stop and look at the monitor, so he paused for just a moment for my heart to regain normal sinus rhythm then he continued with placement of the catheter.

The following days were occupied with scheduling Joanne's forty-eight-hour hospital stay for her pre-transplant workup. On the day of the workup, I took Joanne to St. Michael's Hospital and as I hugged her goodbye I imagined I felt as Sarah did when she had to leave me there. I was very concerned because Joanne had never been hospitalized or had an IV.

The results of Joanne's pre-transplant workup were excellent. She was perfectly healthy and exhibited no signs of PKD or any other type of disease. Our last step was the final crossmatch which was negative. This meant less chance of rejecting the transplanted organ (allograft). Once again, I thought how good life is. I should make mention here that Medicare in the State of Florida covered all of Joanne's medical expenses, as is their standard practice when dealing with donor's without medical insurance.

Since Joanne's test results were all favorable, we set the date for the transplant, Saturday, September 16. I wanted Joanne to know that I was glad that I was the one with PKD and if our roles were reversed there would be no question in my mind as to my obligation toward her. I felt the same way she did and giving her one of my kidneys would have been the only course available to me.

We had a week to wait and plan. During which time, Joanne jokingly said that along with her kidney, I would probably inherit her thick curly hair and craving for certain types of foods and coffee. Neither of us knew at the time just how right she was, especially with respect to the cravings.

Wednesday, before the surgery, we went to the Transplant Center and the hospital to pre-register and we were told that the Center had an offer of a kidney for me. A crossmatch was done but Joanne's kidney was a better match so the center did not consider making me a formal offer of the kidney. Meanwhile, Joanne and I went shopping for loose fitting clothes to wear during the weeks of recovery after our respective surgeries.

Fanny, another dear friend and co-worker, assumed the lead role and coordinated what each of my co-workers would be doing to help my sister and myself. She also volunteered to take care of my apartment, plants and mail. Since I was in the midst of preparing to move, I also wanted to complete as much of the packing as possible before my transplant. As part of our preparation before the transplant Joanne and I cleaned the refrigerator, disposed of the trash, put clean sheets on the beds and packed our bags.

On the morning of the transplant, Sarah and Katy both arrived at my apartment at 5:30 a.m. to take Joanne and myself to St. Michael's hospital. Upon arriving at the hospital, we were instructed to enter the hospital through the emergency entrance. We were escorted to a changing room where Joanne and I were instructed to change into hospital gowns and await the surgical teams. Joanne and I were very grateful that we were allowed to keep our socks on since it was extremely cold in the changing room. Sarah and Katy were allowed to wait with us and we, all four, were in great spirits. The jokes were flying fast and furious. In fact, there was so much laughter I was surprised we were not reprimanded.

Dr. Taber, who would be harvesting Joanne's kidney, arrived and said that we needed to capture the moment on film. He quickly produced his camera and asked Joanne and myself to strike a pose. The photograph was taken. We were now immortalized wearing identical hospital gowns, matching white socks and no makeup. I hoped most fervently that it was not for publication. With a nod of his head, Dr. Taber motioned for us to follow him, "Walk this way" he said, as he sauntered down the hallway. We were all laughing as we followed Dr. Taber in single file. You would think we were all going for ice cream.

We entered the OR preparation room and the team immediately began working on Joanne. First, the resident, Dr. Andrew Danielson, did the pre-operative history and physical. Then the anesthesiologist administered an epidural, and then the IV. A nurse helped her put on the TED elastic hose.

We talked and laughed for approximately half an hour, as we waited for Joanne to be taken to the OR. When they came for her, we shared a few last minute hugs and kisses before she was wheeled into the OR. As she disappeared through the set of double doors leading to the OR, Joanne executed her best "Lady Diana" wave. She smiled and said, "See you in recovery." It was only then that I began experiencing some anxiety.

I remember saying a silent prayer that Joanne would be alright and that she would not be bothered by any ill effects of the surgery in the future.

During the weeks prior to the surgery, neither Joanne nor myself experienced any anxiety or concern over the impending transplant. In fact, we were both quite excited and looking forward to what we considered an awesome experience.

Katy and Sarah talked about Joanne. They thought it was wonderful to have her with us and what a selfless act she was performing by giving me a kidney. I could not hold back the tears. I thought how lucky I was to have a sister who would endure major surgery and the loss of an organ so I could have a chance at a new life. What a precious gift I had in a sister such as Joanne.

The resident came back to let us know that everything was going well. Dr. Lawrence Rowan, the second surgeon who would be transplanting Joanne's kidney, came to meet me. Closely following him was the resident, Dr. Danielson, the anesthesiologist, and the nurse who all followed the same procedure as they had done with Joanne. Fanny arrived in time to join Katy and Sarah as they were wishing me well. So, with one last hug and kiss, I was wheeled into the OR.

During our surgeries, Sarah, Katy and Fanny waited anxiously for news as to how the surgeries were progressing. Dr. Danielson made frequent trips from the OR to the waiting room to keep my friends apprised of our progress.

Two hours later Joanne's surgery was over and she was taken to the recovery room. My surgery continued. Joanne looked at the clock on the wall each time she awoke, and each time it was 20-30 minutes later. Five hours had gone by and there was still no sign of me. Considering the surgery was supposed to be two to three hours in duration, Joanne and my friends became concerned. I was told that Sarah, in her concern, paced the floor and straightened all the pictures hanging in the waiting room.

Finally, I was brought into the recovery room and Joanne and my friends were allowed to see me. Sarah said that she could tell that something was not right or had gone wrong because I looked as though every drop of blood had been drained from my body. She said that my head except for my face was wrapped in white bandages and completely obscured my hair, and she could not tell where my lips were because I was so pale.

She immediately questioned one of the surgeons, asking why I looked so badly. His response was that I had just endured major surgery. Sarah, persistent person that she is, countered by saying that she had seen many people after they had experienced major surgery and they never looked as badly as I did. They at least had some color in their faces.

On the drive home, Sarah told Katy that despite the doctor's denials, she was certain that something had in fact gone wrong. I myself only remember hearing that the surgery had gone well. Katy touched my hand and said that it was all over. Sarah was smiling down at me and she kept passing her hand over my head and cheek. I could not keep my eyes open. I remember smiling because it was over and I was grateful to see familiar smiling faces. When I tried to speak, my throat was very dry and sore from being intubated, and the only thing I said was, "Too much pain, too much pain, more drugs." Everyone left and Joanne and I remained in the recovery room till the following morning then we were moved to intensive care, where we spent the following day.

Dr. Rowan came to my room the following morning to tell me that I needed to be transfused. That was the last thing I expected to hear. Apparently, I had sustained a great deal of blood loss during surgery and my hemoglobin and hematocrit were dangerously low. He then said they were all concerned because they could not understand why I would not stop bleeding. Nowhere in my medical record did it mention the possibility of my having a bleeding disorder.

I could not believe what I was hearing. My heart sank. I knew in an instant what had gone wrong. I said to the surgeon, "I know what happened, the concentrated 500 Heparin® was not aspirated from both ports of my Quinton® catheter before the IV was attached. I believe the Heparin® anticoagulated my entire blood supply".

My body was already being sensitized by my sisters antigens causing the formation of antibodies. I was concerned about the effect the transfusion would have on my body, because of the introduction of additional antigens, which would elevate my Patient Reactive Antibody (PRA) level. This could make me a difficult match if I ever needed another kidney transplant.

I continued to feel weak, my voice was barely a whisper and I was exhausted. I was told that I would feel much better after I was transfused with four pints of blood. Joanne on the other hand was extremely nauseous. She could not open her mouth to speak without throwing up.

They wheeled Joanne by so I could see her and I asked her how she felt, she simply gave me the thumbs down sign. In that moment I experienced a tremendous wave of guilt.

Dr. Danielson kept a close watch on us. He determined that Joanne was allergic to the Morphine® which was continually being administered by the epidural. The epidural was removed and she was given an anti-emetic, Compazine®, which did not have any effect. Phenergan® was then administered and she at once began to experience relief from her nausea, and was able to consume and keep down clear liquids.

A sense of awe and wonder came over me. I placed my hand over the area where Joanne's kidney was lying in my abdomen. It was amazing to me that I had an organ functioning in me which only hours before was functioning in my sister. The feeling was unbelievable.

My sense of awe was put on pause when I saw my scar for the first time. I was shocked. It was not what I had expected. It was ugly and extended from across my pubic area and curved up along the right side of my abdomen almost to my waist in a semi-circle. I do not remember how many stitches or clamps there were, I only remember that there were numerous. I wondered if the scar could be seen if I wore a bathing suit.

Joanne was making a remarkable recovery. She was able to walk in a relatively short period of time. This being so, she was able to visit me frequently from her room next door. Her recovery was attributed to the fact that she is ten years younger than I am and she was healthy from the beginning.

Because Joanne was always feeling cold and I was always very warm she frequently climbed into bed with me to keep warm. We would eat together, watch TV together, our friends would visit us together and the nurses would take our vital signs together. All the nurses would comment on how cute we both looked. We felt like kids on a sleep-over.

CHAPTER ELEVEN

POST TRANSPLANT MEDICATIONS

> *Good movies make you care,*
> *make you believe in possibilities again.*
>
> -Pauline Kael

Since I was so weak Dr. Taber did not have me get out of bed and walk on the day after surgery. He waited until the second day, until I had been transfused and felt stronger. When I attempted to stand, my ankles continually buckled under my weight, even with a nurse on each side for support. I was still too weak. We gave up and decided to try again the following day.

Joanne's kidney was working very well. In Dr. Taber's vernacular he told Joanne, "Your sister is peeing like a race horse." Thank heavens for Foley® catheters because I could not stand up under my own steam let alone manage numerous trips to the bathroom. I kept the nurses aides busy emptying the urine from the bag at the other end of my Foley® catheter, and the tissue fluid and blood from my Jackson-Pratt® catheter.

During one of Sarah's visits to the hospital, Joanne was lying in bed with me. Hugo Bianco, the kidney patient from across the hall also came to visit, bringing with him his IV bag which he hung on the pole attached to my bed. Chad Evans another kidney patient, not hospitalized at that time, also came to visit. A nurse came in to check vital signs, took a look around the room, looked at the chart he was carrying and finally in exasperation asked, "Alright, which one of you is the patient?" We all raised our hands and began to laugh. Once the laughter subsided I finally admitted to being the patient he was seeking.

Dr. Taber came in next and was surprised to find four of his patients together. I invited him to join us saying that we were having a support group meeting and that the pizza and Pepsi® would be arriving shortly. This of course was only in jest.

The following day, Joanne and I were moved to isolation to remove us from the hospital environment. This was done to reduce the risk of infection to me because of my immunosuppression (the prevention of formation of the immune response). After all, hospitals are filled with "sick people" and was not a good place to be in my weakened state. The immunosuppression medication decimates the T-cells (first response cells of your immune system) to an acceptably low level to avoid rejection of the transplanted kidney.

While in isolation, I could not make any long-distance telephone calls, so I gave Sarah and Katy a list of certain family members and friends I needed them to telephone on Joanne's and my behalf. I also asked them to convey the message that Joanne and I would be telephoning once we were out of isolation.

The transplant coordinator, John Crawford, came to see me carrying with him a list of all the medications I would be taking. I knew that there would be quite a few, but nineteen!!! The list of medications included: Acetaminophen®, Acyclovir®, Imuran®, Tums®, Sandimmune® (cyclosporin), OKT3® via IV infusion once a day for the first 5-7 days post transplantation, Nystatin® swish and swallow, Nu-Iron®, Prednisone®, Zantac®, Bactrim®, Neutra-Phos®, Percocet® for pain, Zovirax®, Amphosec® liquid, Dipyri lamole®, Promethazine®, and Phenergan® for nausea.

I read all the literature I was provided on my medications paying particular attention to the contraindications and I learned that these medications could produce problems with impotency and lack of sex drive in men. Many female transplant patients may experience a lack of sex drive and/or irregular periods. Some may be infertile but others may be able to conceive. The immunosuppressant medications could also produce mood swings, alteration of personality, loss or increase of appetite, weight gain, and excessive loss or growth of hair. The strength and combination of these medications are the equivalent of chemotherapy. Many of the complications developed by transplant patients are drug-related and not organ-specific.

I kept my medications in a row on the kitchenette counter according to the order in which they were listed in the manila folder. Before each meal, I read off the names and dosages of the medications, while Joanne, dispensed the medications into a cup according to their respective dosages.

The number of tablets was overwhelming, therefore my meals were punctuated by the taking of medications. Each time I felt the need to take a drink, I would consume a few of the tablets. This was my way of taking my medications and avoiding filling up, while leaving room for my meals.

My least favorite was the Sandimmune® (cyclosporin) because it had an awful smell and taste, and I had a difficult time keeping it down. My second least favorite was the OKT3® which was administered via IV or a butterfly in the back of the hand. This medication produced night sweats, fevers, chills, headaches and an excruciating amount of joint pain. The night sweats produced by the OKT3® were terrible. Joanne had to help me strip the bed of all its sheets and replace them, along with my socks and gown, because they would become drenched in sweat. This became our nightly ritual. It was awful waking in the middle of the night freezing, experiencing chills, and soaking wet. However, it was just as awful waking in the morning and not being able to move because of severe joint pain.

Our morning ritual consisted of Joanne helping me out of bed to a chair and placing wet warm wash cloths on my neck, shoulders, elbows, wrists, knees and ankles to warm them and ease the joint pain. This ritual took about an hour. It was during these moments when I could hardly move that I questioned whether the transplant was worth it. I questioned also, if I would ever again feel normal, healthy, or pain free. With our morning washcloth ritual observed, we prepared ourselves for our daily doctor's appointment.

I was always weighed at the beginning of each visit. In one week's time my weight increased from 120-138 pounds. Since I was not eating as much as Dr. Taber would like, I could only assume this weight gain was "bloat" brought on by the use of the steroids, specifically the Prednisone®. So here I was, face and body swollen, body scarred and feeling hideous. As one of my friends put it, "I felt as though I fell from the top of an ugly tree and hit every branch on the way down." Because I bled during surgery, my abdomen was distended and leaking tissue fluid which was pink-tinged but odorless and clear. The leak was so profuse, that Joanne and I were constantly changing my dressing. This went on all day and night. While I was waiting to see the transplant coordinator on one of our visits to Dr. Taber's office, I began to leak. I hoped that I would be ushered into an examination room before my clothes became fluid-soaked.

John, the transplant coordinator, came to usher me in, and as soon as I stood up a stream of fluid began running down my leg. By the time I had taken three steps the fluid had already reached my ankle. As if by magic, John produced some gauze for me to mop-up the fluid, just before it reached my sock. The leak of fluid continued through one more night then ceased.

Joanne got a clean bill of health. Aside from a nagging cough and a few twinges around her incision, she was doing very well. Her incision measured 4-5 inches and left a fine line on the right side of her waist. Dr. Taber does not believe in removing a rib in order to remove a donor kidney. This type of incision is referred to as a "subcostal lateral flank incision without rib resection." This causes less stress, less pain, and a quicker recovery time.

CHAPTER TWELVE

LOSING MY SISTER'S KIDNEY

> *Life has, indeed, many ills, but the mind that views every*
> *object in its most cheering aspect, and every doubtful dispensation*
> *as replete with latent good, bears within itself a powerful*
> *and perpetual antidote.*
>
> **-Lydia H. Sigourney**

For the first three days in isolation our meals were being delivered from the hospital, therefore, we did not have to concern ourselves with food preparation. Our friends also brought us fruits and lots of other good things to eat. We had enough food to feed an army. As prescribed, after my morning meal, I took an antacid (Amphogel®), and after every meal, I used (Nystatin®) "swish and swallow." This medication was administered by taking a sip, thoroughly rinsing my mouth, then swallowing. Once the medication was swallowed I was not allowed to eat or drink anything for at least five minutes. This medication protects the immunosuppressed patient from acquiring a yeast (thrush) infection in the mouth, throat, and esophagus. This type of infection is extremely painful and inhibits swallowing. I also had to keep a record of the frequency at which I urinated. Joanne and I were both amazed to see that in a 24 hour period I urinated an unbelievable 23 times.

While still in isolation, Sarah and Katy came to visit us one afternoon after work. As they shared the events of their day, Joanne and I both sat each holding a pillow to our incisions to minimize our discomfort while laughing. As they were leaving, Katy observed an artificial plant just outside the front door of our room. She said that it looked like a marijuana plant and she hoped that she would not see the plant stripped of all its leaves on her next visit. We all laughed and said good night.

As soon as Sarah and Katy were out of sight, Joanne and I, while laughing, dragged the plant inside our room and hid it in a corner and anxiously awaited Katy's return to see if she would notice its absence. Two days later, Katy came to visit and we were not disappointed because her first words were, "Where is the plant?" I might add that many of our friends could not visit us in isolation because they had small children or had recently been sick or vaccinated.

On Friday, six days post transplantation, Joanne's and my stitches and clamps would be removed and we could both go home either Saturday or Sunday. We opted for Saturday because Joanne was experiencing some depression, and we were both suffering from cabin fever. Fanny volunteered to take us home. When she arrived, we were both dressed, packed and ready to go. As always, Fanny brought her camera to capture the moment on film.

After a few photographs were taken of Joanne and myself striking various poses, we took a long last look around what had become our second home. Joanne and Fanny quickly loaded the van and we were off. It was good to feel the sunlight on my face and arms and feel the wind blowing through my hair. I felt as though all my senses were heightened and everything I saw looked new to me, even colors seemed brighter than I remembered. Freedom at last.

We arrived at my apartment and were welcomed by a musty smell, but it was wonderful to us. Joanne opened the sliding doors to the screened patio to air the apartment. Fanny meanwhile helped us unpack and put our belongings away. Now we could get back to enjoying home cooking, cable television and familiar surroundings. Fanny made sure that our prescriptions were filled and bought us hamburgers for lunch, so I could satisfy my cravings.

Fanny left after Joanne and I were through eating. I told Joanne that when she was back home in Trinidad and I felt lonely I could reach down and touch her kidney and I would feel as though she was with me. Each time I touched her kidney it would give her the feeling that someone was tickling her side.

Sunday night, I awoke at 11:45 p.m., with a throbbing pain over the area of my allograft. The pain was so severe-that it took my breath away. I removed my clothing, took two Percocet® and paced the floor rubbing my incision. Forty minutes later, the pain had not subsided so I placed a telephone call to Rosemary, the transplant coordinator on-call that night. When she returned my call I relayed my symptoms.

Rosemary said that I should wait a little longer for the Percocet® to take effect. I asked if I could use a heating pad. She replied that a heating pad was allowed since a week had elapsed since my surgery. In retrospect, I realize this was a situation when the patient should have taken control of the situation and proceeded directly to the ER. I could not conceive that anything could possibly be wrong, plus the fact that my decision making process was impaired by the effects of the Percocet®. I got back in bed and applied the heating pad to my incision. An hour later I began experiencing relief and was able to sleep. I awoke the following morning without the throbbing pain. One sore spot remained and it hurt only when touched. Joanne and I then went to our regularly scheduled appointment with Dr. Taber.

I gave a detailed account of the events of the previous night and the opinion was that I probably had a build-up of fluid. Dr. Taber left the room and returned bearing a syringe with a very long needle and before I could ask his intentions he inserted the needle into my abdomen just above the incision as though he was throwing a dart.

I sat wide-eyed in amazement both by the method of inserting the needle and the fact that I did not feel any pain. I attributed the fact that I did not feel any pain to the incision still being numb from surgery and the effect of the Percocet®. Dr. Taber pulled on the plunger but did not aspirate any fluid. He then removed the needle, said I looked great, and sent me on my way.

After lunch Fanny came to take Joanne and myself on a two-hour shopping trip. I felt as though I was a normal person enjoying a normal everyday activity. It was great to be free of tubes, needles, shunts and accesses. The only thing I missed was the adjustable hospital bed because it was easy to get in and out of. We stopped for lunch, then returned home.

Joanne went to the kitchen to get a drink and I went to the bedroom to change my clothes. Just as I finished undressing, the phone rang. It was Rosemary. She said that my laboratory results were very bad, either the kidney was not function-ing or I was experiencing a massive rejection episode. I was instructed to pro-ceed directly to the ER at St. Michael's Hospital and that Dr. Taber would meet me there.

I sat on the edge of my bed and began to cry, I had only just begun to enjoy my new-found freedom. After all I had been through, I hoped that I was not losing my kidney (allograft). I called to Joanne and she came running into the bedroom. I quickly explained the situation, then I telephoned Sarah and Katy and asked for a ride to the hospital. Sarah said she would be at my apartment in fifteen minutes to take us to the hospital. Katy would meet us there.

I made a conscious effort to think positively and decided not to worry until I knew what was the matter. I felt very well and could not believe that anything was wrong. We arrived at the ER and was whisked to the Radiology Department where a physician performed a renal scan using radioactive contrast. The scan clearly revealed my native kidneys but did not reveal my allograft.

Dr. Taber walked in, already wearing his surgical garb. After a quick look at the monitor he advised me that exploratory surgery would be required. He needed to actually see the allograft to determine the cause of the problem. Once again, my sister and my friends were concerned. As I was being wheeled to the OR, I asked them to call several of my friends and family to inform them of my situation. Dr. Taber anxiously paced the floor, as the anesthesiologist made several attempts before he could secure an IV in the back of my left hand. Dr. Taber said he was relieved to hear that I felt well, that meant there was hope. I looked at him and said, "Whatever the outcome, I know that you will do your best for me." The last things I remember before being wheeled into the OR, was Joanne telling me not to worry, and Sarah's concerned look and tears in her eyes.

I awoke in the recovery room with the familiar dry sore throat and pain emanating from the right side of my abdomen. I also felt pain in my right subclavicular area (below the clavicle/collar bone). I had a difficult time staying awake and my eyelids felt heavy due to the after effects of the anesthesia. In one of my lucid moments I saw Dr. Taber looking down at me and he said the words I will never forget, "We lost the kidney, we could not get it to work, we had to remove it." I had a sickening feeling in the pit of my stomach. I was devastated not only for myself but also for Joanne who had endured major surgery and the loss of a major organ, all for nothing. Then a horrible thought occurred to me, I had to return to hemodialysis and anxiety attacks. Mercifully, darkness descended upon me again as I fell asleep.

The following morning I awoke to discover that the cause of the pain in my right subclavian area was from an access for hemodialysis which was placed immediately after the loss of the kidney. Dr. Taber then entered my room with his shoulders hunched, head hung low, and a sense of intense sadness on his face. He could barely look me in the eyes. He expressed his deep sense of regret for my loss and told me that he removed the kidney, flushed it with UM solution and reattached it anattempt to restore it to working order, but it was to no avail.

As I remember, he said that the transplanted kidney's artery clotted at the point of the anastomosis (an end-to-end union of two vessels) to my artery. He did not know if it was a technical error on their part such as a loose stitch, or something physical on my part, e.g. allergy to the suture material or underlying health problem, which caused the kidney to clot. He would have more information for me after the pathology was performed on the kidney. Several days later, the pathology revealed, "...no evidence of immunologic reaction or a rejection." The true reason for the loss of my allograft still managed to elude my physicians.

Dr. Taber said that the entire surgical team took the loss of the kidney personally. I felt as though I should say something to comfort him, and he looked at me in astonishment as I said, "I know that you did your best for me. I am going to be alright." He then left my room and I laid in bed anxiously awaiting Joanne's arrival. With a sense of resignation and defeat, I wondered how I was going to face Joanne and what words of comfort I could offer. I felt a huge sense of guilt, depression and anger welling up within me. I had begun the mourning process associated with the loss of an organ. To me, it was as real, painful, and devastating a process as mourning the loss of a loved one.

CHAPTER THIRTEEN

RETURNING TO HEMODIALYSIS

*You have to accept what comes and the only important thing
is that you meet it with the best you have to give.*

-Eleanor Roosevelt

I heard a knock on the door and looked up as Dr. Rowan entered my room. He too expressed his disappointment at the loss of the allograft. He further stated that Dr. Taber was most disappointed at his inability to save Joanne's kidney.

Later, when Joanne arrived she came over to me immediately and gave me a hug. I could not hold back the tears. I expressed what I was feeling and once the tears subsided Joanne told me that she had done all her crying the night before and given a lot of thought to what she would say to me. "This situation is just between the two of us" she said, "the kidney was my gift to you." "Everything happens for a reason. Can you imagine how badly I would have felt had we not tried the transplant? As far as I am concerned its over. If it does not bother me, it should not bother you."

What a sister! Everyone should have one like her. I had always thought of Joanne as exceptional and there had always been a special bond between us, but the transplant brought us even closer together. What Joanne did for me is definitely a demonstration of unconditional love. It takes someone with an extraordinary amount of love and compassion to make such a sacrifice.

Hemodialysis at St. Michael's Hospital was a horrible ordeal. I did not want to be there. I experienced a severe anxiety attack and insisted on not being left alone. I had to have someone holding my hand. Somehow it made me feel grounded and also made enduring the treatment possible. Nurses held my hand in shifts. Finally, the mother of one of the other hemodialysis patients was asked to hold my hand until my sister arrived.

Joanne's daily visits were the high points of my days. Not only was it wonderful to have her with me but she brought with her my favorite ham sandwich made on Boston hard rolls. After only two hemodialysis treatments my right subclavian access clotted and had to be replaced. Dr. Rowan was going to perform the replacement of the access. This is the same resident whose visits I enjoyed because of his wonderful sense of humor. That day, not only was I not laughing, but I was not looking forward to seeing him.

He entered my room with two nurses in attendance who positioned themselves on either side of my bed and proceeded to take hold of my hands. I realized then that I was in for a rough ride. Dr. Rowan revealed a rather large syringe with a very long needle. The presence of the nurses became clear. He proceeded to insert the needle in my right subclavian area. I was amazed by the sight of the needle disappearing into my body. There were a few seconds delay before I felt the intense pain as the Lidocaine® was being injected. Dr. Rowan and the nurses then left the room, returning in approximately 15 minutes, allowing the Lidocaine® to take effect. A sterile drape was strategically placed, and the resident cut and removed the stitches holding the old catheter in place, and inserted a guide wire down the opening.

In one very swift motion the old catheter was removed and the new one was slipped into position over the guide wire, then the guide wire was removed and the new catheter was stitched in place. Through the pain, I vaguely remember telling Dr. Rowan that he was lucky that I held him in high esteem, otherwise his life would be in peril.

I now had to face my return to the Dialysis Center for my treatments, a place I thought I would never see again. I experienced what I could only term as "dread." I had a difficult enough time accepting hemodialysis before the transplant, now I was angry that I had to be there, and felt as though I should not be going through this again. I should now be enjoying a sense of freedom and well-being.

My first hemodialysis treatment at the Dialysis Center brought with it the worst of my anxiety attacks. As we pulled into the parking lot of the Center, I could feel my jaw and stomach muscles tensing. I entered the Center with a sullen face and shoulders hung low, exhibiting the resignation that I was feeling as I walked slowly toward one of the nurses to inquire about my seat assignment.

Once I was in my seat I could feel myself becoming more and more anxious. A short time after I was connected to the hemodialysis machine I became very agitated. I could feel the muscles in my arms, legs and abdomen contracting to the point that I experienced physical pain.

In an attempt to control my agitation, I ate crackers and fruit and even attempted to read. I did manage to sleep for brief moments but my sleep was continually interrupted by the nurses checking my blood pressure. Each time I would awaken to the harsh reality of my situation and watching my blood enter and exit the machine did nothing to alleviate my agitation. After one of these occasions, I began experiencing restless legs and arms. I began to shift restlessly in my seat and looked at my watch to find that I had been in treatment for only one hour. The fact that I still had two hours of dialysis remaining was my undoing.

My stomach muscles became extremely tense and I wanted to get out of the recliner and walk around. I was not allowed to do this because movement impeded the flow of blood through the Quinton® catheter. I then experienced a huge sense of panic and began pulling on the tubing as though I was disconnecting myself from the hemodialysis machine. My sister Joanne called to a nurse for help. The nurse who came to our aid tried to calm me down by having me look in her eyes while taking deep slow breaths.

She quietly said, "In through the nose, out through the mouth." After several deep breaths I experienced a sense of calm. The sense of calm was short lived because within a few minutes I could feel my body tensing once again. My agitation became more intense with every passing moment. I felt the need to look Joanne in the eyes to keep myself from experiencing total panic. While looking Joanne in the eyes, I held her hands tightly in mine, while in a soothing voice, she continuously uttered nurturing and supportive words. So intense was my anxiety that I would not allow her to look away or release my hands. We maintained that awkward position for the remaining two hours of my treatment. Joanne must have been exhausted. I was never more grateful to have her with me. Without her there, they would have had to sedate me.

Subsequent to my first dialysis treatment, I began researching (RLS) Restless Legs Syndrome and discovered that RLS is a medical condition which affects the legs or arms. RLS can affect those afflicted when they are sitting, lying or especially at bedtime. RLS can be painful and can occur during sleeping or waking hours. The pain, creepy, crawley, pulling or gnawing feelings are temporarily relieved by stretching or moving the legs.

RLS can limit the length of time a person can travel by any means of transportation because of their inability to sit still for long periods of time. RLS can also inhibit a person's ability to enjoy various types of entertainment e.g., plays and movies, or attend meetings. This can all lead to anxiety and/or depression.

The majority of RLS cases are caused by: poor circulation in the legs, nerve problems, muscle disorders, kidney disease, alcoholism, and mineral or vitamin deficiencies. Other triggering factors are: stopping or starting medications, fatigue, smoking, caffeine, prolonged exposure to very warm or coldweather.

Some home remedies which can provide relief are: hot baths, leg massages, ice packs, heating pad, aspirin, pain relievers, exercise, or elimination of caffeine. Some patients have experienced relief with the use of Vitamin E or calcium, although there is no scientific data to support this claim.

In preparation for my future dialysis treatments, I was forced to return to my old regimen of 2.5 mg of Xanax® and 325 mg of Percocet® one half hour prior to treatment in order to sleep through the entire process.

Being stuck with those large needles for dialysis was very painful. I tried a topical anesthetic several times over the area where the needles would be inserted. Not only did it not anesthetize the area, but it left me with a very red blotch.

On my next appointment at the Dialysis Center, all the patients, myself included, were switched to a new and improved F-80® artificial kidney, to be used during dialysis treatments. The fibers within the artificial kidney were made of a new and more efficient fiber which was believed to improve filtration, produce less side effects, and make the treatments more tolerable for the patients.

After my first treatment with the F-80® artificial kidney, I experienced an increase in temperature, achy joints, chills, nausea, a rash, and a headache of migraine proportion. All my instincts told me that it was an allergic reaction to the F-80® artificial kidney.

I reported my list of symptoms to my dialysis nurse, and to confirm my suspicions, I decided to have a second treatment with the F-80® kidney to see if I would experience the same symptoms again.

After my second treatment, I did in fact experience all the same symptoms and this time I reported them to my nephrologist. I asked him to write me a prescription to use the older model artificial kidney to rule out the possibility of an allergic reaction. I had my next dialysis treatment with the older model artificial kidney and I did not experience any of the symptoms I had previously. Consequently, I was switched back to the older model artificial kidney from that time forward. This was a classic example that all things do not work for all people.

CHAPTER FOURTEEN

DEPRESSION

*Let me remember that each life must follow its own course,
and that what happens to other people has absolutely
nothing to do with what happens to me.*

-Marjorie Holmes

It was mid November and I had hoped that I would be fully recovered and able to participate in the craft show. The crafters were in the process of delivering their wares to Sarah's home and I mustered what little energy I could, and together with Joanne, Sarah and Katy, and other friends, we priced hundreds of items for the show. Joanne, being the artist that she is, hand painted the sign bearing our company name. We spent many hours working late into the night and wee hours of the morning, arranging and decorating Sarah's home in preparation for the show.

Finally, we were ready and the Saturday of the craft show arrived. This was also a dialysis day for me. Joanne took me to the show after dialysis, but I felt so badly I was only able to stay for two hours before I had to be taken home, fed, and put to bed. I was told that at the close of our first day we sold $900 worth of craft items. The second day, I felt much better and was able to spend the entire time with my friends. Unfortunately, we did not make very much money that day.

Remember the old saying, "After joy comes sorrow," well, once the excitement of the show had abated, we were left with "grim reality," otherwise known as the "clean-up process."

Sarah and Katy took charge of returning the unsold craft items to the crafters together with the money they made at the show. Also, Sarah's home had to be returned to its former condition. So much was involved with putting on a show that we were not sure if we ever wanted to venture in those waters again.

By now, I had come to terms with the fact that I had to be back on dialysis. I was having a difficult time with the many Quinton® catheter exchanges I was forced to endure because of clotting. Consequently, I spent a great deal of time in in the hospital. Dr. Thornton thought that all things considered I was doing very well. He said, "You never look as though you have anything wrong with you." I replied, "Because I always take great pains with my appearance." He also said, "Your possibility of receiving sympathy would be greatly increased if you stopped wearing makeup." I think my nephrologist was a frustrated comedian.

Among the many issues discussed, was my need for placement of a permanent access for hemodialysis. He insisted that we set a date for the surgery. This time the vascular surgeon would place a straight Gortex® graft in my left lower arm from inside my left wrist to my antecubital fossa (bend in the arm opposite the elbow).

To attain the permanent access, I was admitted to the St. Ignatius Hospital for a 23-hour stay. The orderly recognized me because I worked at the facility. As we entered the holding area, the orderly announced that he was wheeling in a VIP. I saw the familiar faces of the ER nurses and the anesthesiologists. They recognized me on sight and remembered my name asking, "So, Donna, what are we doing for you today." It occurred to me that I had been spending too much time in the OR because I was on first name terms with the anesthesiologists. "Take a deep breath" was the last thing I remembered hearing before waking up in the recovery room.

When I awoke, I became aware of the surgeon's face looking down at me. "The surgery went well," he said. He added that placement was difficult because my veins were very small. Again, I felt a huge amount of pain emanating from the area of my left wrist and inside my left elbow. Once again I relied on Percocet® for pain relief. I left the hospital with my temporary access in place as a precautionary measure. After my permanent access was used twice successfully the temporary access was removed. Unfortunately, after only six weeks of use my permanent access clotted.

My luck was running true to form. The first week in December, I was again admitted to the hospital to have a vascular surgeon remove the clot from my access to restoring it to working order. For this reason, Dr. Thornton held the placement of yet another temporary access in abeyance. I was especially grateful for this because the access would be placed in my right femoral vein (right groin just above the thigh).

Joanne took me to the hospital at 6 a.m., the morning of the surgery for what was supposed to be a twenty-three-hour stay. I sent her home to sleep promising to call her from my room once I had recovered from surgery. When I awoke in my room I was told that the clot was removed and I was placed on Coumadin® anticoagulation therapy. Twenty-four hours later my permanent access clotted again, and the vascular surgeon was summoned to remove the clot in a second attempt to save the access. Before my second trip to the OR, however, I was taken to the Dialysis Center for placement of a temporary access.

Dr. Thornton and his resident, Dr. Ira Gordon, a nephrology resident, arrived shortly after I did. Much to my chagrin, Dr. Gordon placed himself on my right side and Dr. Thornton stood on my left giving him instructions. I knew I was in trouble.

Dr. Gordon uncovered and shaved my right groin area. He then cleaned the area with Betadyne® and injected it with Lidocaine®. I had been injected with Lidocaine® many times in the past but it never hurt as much as it did that morning. After waiting several minutes for the Lidocaine® to take affect, Dr. Gordon approached me again, this time carrying my instrument of torture, the Quinton® catheter.

At the instruction of Dr. Thornton, Dr. Gordon attempted to locate my femoral vein which runs parallel to the femoral artery and lies adjacent to it. The easiest way to accomplish this is to locate my femoral pulse, which he did.

I was not prepared for the pain which resulted as Dr. Gordon inserted the access. He missed the vein on his first, second, third, and fourth attempts and hit the artery instead, which caused a profuse amount of cherry red blood to erupt from the puncture site and collected in a pool on the bedclothes under my right thigh. As he wiggled the access in an attempt to locate the vein, it caused an enormous amount of pain.

By now, the Lidocaine® was wearing off and the pain from my right groin area was severe. I gritted my teeth and could feel my temper rising. I then cast my eyes heavenward and wondered how much more I was expected to endure. Finally, Dr. Thornton traded places with Dr. Gordon and attempted to place the access himself. Mercifully, he managed to place it on his first attempt, but not after he had to wiggle the access a little himself. Once placed, Dr. Thornton traded places with Dr. Gordon again and instructed him to stitch the catheter in place.

The benefit of the Lidocaine® was now nonexistent. I asked for more to be administered and was told that they were almost through and once through, I would be given some Percocet®. I felt the sting of the needle piercing my skin and also felt the suture material being pulled through my skin and tied. In that moment I dubbed Dr. Gordon "The Barbarian."

The stinging and burning from the placement of the sutures continued, along with excruciating and throbbing pain emanating from the access in my right groin. I was very angry. I had visions of castrating Dr. Gordon with my long fingernails, without the use of Lidocaine®!

My sister entered the cubicle with the curtains which now opened and with one look at my face she could tell that I was not happy. Her first words to me were,

"I can see that it did not go well. You look really angry." I nodded my head in ascent. At my sister's words, Dr. Gordon paused from writing in my chart and quickly looked up at me then at my sister, and just as quickly and self-consciously looked down again, burying his head in my chart. I then gratefully accepted the two Percocet® the dialysis nurse brought me.

After waiting a while for the Percocet® to take effect, the nurse began my dialysis treatment. I slept for several hours and by the time I awoke my treatment was almost over. Shortly thereafter, I was returned to my room where I remained as motionless as I could to avoid exacerbation of my right groin pain. Because of the position of the access, I could not bend my leg at the top of the thigh, which would allow me to sit erect. I was also not allowed to get out of bed or attempt to walk without someone in attendance. A "fall precaution" sign was placed on the door outside my room.

My stay in the hospital was made bearable by a mixture concocted by my sister. This concoction consisted of vegetarian vegetable soup, tomato soup, lots of potatoes and whole kernel corn. I enjoyed this piping hot concoction to such an extent that I insisted on having it for dinner every night.

The following day, I was taken down to the OR again to remove the clot from my fistula. The clot was removed and twenty-four hours later it clotted again. The following morning brought the same scenario which was a last ditch attempt to remove the new clot from my fistula. If this attempt failed, the vascular surgeon would immediately proceed with placement of yet another permanent access in my left upper arm. When I awoke after surgery, the surgeon told me that he removed the clot from the straight fistula in my left lower arm.

As he was suturing my arm, he actually witnessed the clot forming again. He then removed the entire fistula and sutured the wound, then immediately proceeded with placement of a fistula in my left upper arm, in the hope that it would be successful.

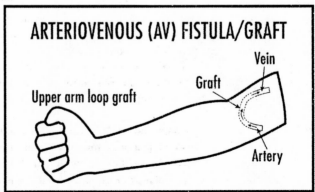

ARTERIOVENOUS (AV) FISTULA/GRAFT

Vein

Graft

Upper arm loop graft

Artery

The pain now emanating from my left upper arm rivaled the pain I was experiencing in my right groin, and it was intensified with the minimum of movement. I looked down at my bandaged left upper arm and it seemed to be three to four times its normal size. I could only assume that the bandages accounted for this illusion. The constant throbbing in my left upper arm was so excruciating that once again I requested Percocet® for pain relief.

That night, I shifted and felt as though I was lying down in a pool of liquid which extended from my left shoulder down to my hind quarters. I buzzed for the nurse. When she arrived she gently lifted my shoulders off the bed just enough to look behind and saw to her horror that I was lying in a large pool of blood. She summoned help and both my gown and bedclothes were changed and my incision was redressed.

I finally got my first chance to see my left upper arm. I was horrified. My arm had actually swollen to three times its normal size. My shoulder and behind my left arm were especially swollen, and black, because of the pooling of blood from lying down.

I had to keep my left arm immobile. It was placed on a pillow as high as my arm would permit. I felt totally helpless because I could not move my right leg either. I laughed out loud at what a pathetic sight I was. I continued to bleed so profusely, my bandages and bedclothes required changing every two hours, for the following 5 days.

The fistula could not be checked for a bruit until the edema or swelling had subsided. On the fifth day also, believe it or not, I began menstruating. What else could happen to me now, I thought, as I began to laugh in earnest. One should never tempt fate, for as luck would have it, I began feeling very weak and each time I attempted to raise my head off the pillow I felt extremely faint.

On the sixth day, I felt a little better while lying down and got out of bed because I felt an urgent need to use the bathroom. As I reached the bathroom, I felt the all too familiar sensation of feeling cold, then lightheaded, then a sense that blackness was about to descend as I was fainting. I had the presence of mind to grab the string on the emergency alarm and yelled that I was falling. In response to my yell, I heard several pairs of footsteps thundering down the hall. I was determined to return to my bed and not fall on the bathroom floor. I took very slow, deep breaths and began my trip back to my bed.

By the time the nurses entered my room, I had managed to reach my bed and was attempting to climb in. I had made a huge miscalculation. I thought I was strong enough or I would not have attempted to get out of bed. I never attempted anything again without help. I was placed on Heparin® and Coumadin® anticoagulation therapy because the physicians thought this would prevent my new fistula from clotting.

The bleeding together with the anticoagulation therapy lowered my blood pressure to 89/50 mm/Hg, my HGB (hemoglobin) was 7.0 g/dL (normal 12.0-15.5 g/dL) and my PTT (partial thromboplastin time), was 200 seconds (normal 22.7-36.1 seconds). I could not lift my head off the pillow without fear of fainting. To make matters worse, I began experiencing an intense throbbing pain in the area of my right ovary. It became so intense that I could not lie still.

After reporting my symptoms to the nephrologist on call, he ordered the addition of saline to my IV in an attempt to raise my blood pressure. A CT scan was also ordered to determine if I was experiencing any internal bleeding. Several hours later, the nephrologist came to see me with the results. There was no sign of internal bleeding except for a minute amount in the area of my right ovary, indicating the rupture of an ovarian cyst. I felt as though I was in a Shakespearian tragedy or in an episode of the Twilight Zone.

Originally, I was admitted for a twenty-three hour hospital stay, but spent two weeks instead. I felt as though I had checked in for an oil and filter change, but had a complete overhaul instead. I made jokes about my warranty running out and everything that could go wrong with my body, actually was. To this point, I had managed to maintain a positive mental attitude and my sense of humor.

I always felt as though I had to be in control of my emotions. I believed myself a very strong person with a huge amount of inner resources and felt that I could endure anything. You can only get away with this for so long before it catches up with you. Trying to be strong all the time is exhausting. There are life experiences when even strong individuals require help and support. It was time to have another conversation with my Heavenly Father. With my unique brand of humor I told Him that I had asked him repeatedly to "Throw me a crumb," and He had waited so long to do so that a mere crumb would no longer suffice; I needed an entire loaf of bread.

Lately, however, I felt as though I was running on empty and had nothing left with which to fight. I was slipping into that deep dark place called depression, and my quality of life was very poor. I was tired of the constellation of injections, surgeries, medications, and the fact that literally every day brought with it a new challenge. There were actual moments when I was so abjectly miserable that I prayed for death. I actually believed that death would be better than what I was enduring.

In desperation, I telephoned my Bishop and told him that my strength was waning. Being the dutiful man that he is, he rushed to see me in the hospital and we had a long talk. I was enveloped by a sweet sense of peace and the assurance that I would be made whole again. I realized that I was presented with these experiences to help me learn and grow. These experiences were also challenges for everyone who knew me, and they all rose to the occasion whenever I was in a time of need.

I began to look at my challenges from a spiritual aspect, and discovered that I was stronger than the challenges. I already possessed the ability and all the tools required to overcome the challenges that were placed before me. I also discovered that I had a certain element of control of those periods when I lost my focus. I regained my focus and perspective by placing my Heavenly Father first, myself second, family third, then friends, etc.

I came to the realization that my life experiences occurred so that I could grow in the areas in which I was lacking. There have been instances, however, when my lessons were learned in retrospect.

I had to have unconditional love for myself because only through love of self could I experience joy, happiness and laughter. I believed that between my Heavenly Father and myself all things were possible. My burden now seemed lighter, and I was filled with the realization that my spiritual, physical, and emotional lives were intertwined. It is one of those life experiences that cannot be fully explained or understood unless it is actually experienced.

CHAPTER FIFTEEN

PERITONEAL DIALYSIS

Every event in life has a purpose.
There are no coincidences,
only opportunities to learn and be creative.

-Anonymous

Several days later, the swelling and constant pain in my left upper arm had decreased sufficiently to allow examination of the new fistula (Gortex® graft). My luck was running true to form, there was no sign of a thrill or bruit, the fistula had clotted. The following morning I was taken down to the OR again to have the clot removed (thrombectomy) from the fistula. If the clot could not be removed, the surgeon would proceed with placement of a permanent access for peritoneal dialysis. Hemodialysis was no longer considered a viable option for me.

Fanny and Ruby, two of my co-workers, came to see me before my surgery and found me crying. Fanny said that she had always compared me to a Superball® because I had an amazing ability to bounce back from my health challenges. "I have never seen you down to this extent before, you are scaring me," Fanny said, as she went in search of a box of tissues.

I asked Fanny to take my pocket pager with her because I was not allowed to take it with me to the OR. I gave her strict instructions to respond if the pager beeped, and to be sure to accept the kidney on my behalf. In spite of my situation, I laughed at the look on Fanny's face, as I hastened to explain that it was purely in jest.

Once in the recovery room after surgery I awoke to that all too familiar pain. This time I was experiencing the pain in my left upper arm and in my abdominal region. Dr. Thornton came to see me to explain that after the removal of the clot, the surgeon began to stitch the wound, but, as he did so, he could actually see the clot forming again and completely occlude the fistula. I made a mental note to discuss further testing with my nephrologist to rule out a hypercoagulable (clotting) problem. My only option now was peritoneal dialysis, which was not initially considered because Dr. Thornton felt that my abdominal cavity was not large enough to accommodate the quantity of dialysate required for adequate dialysis.

Dr. Thornton at once requested the surgeon to proceeded with placement of the Tenckhoff® catheter (a permanent access for peritoneal dialysis). At this point, no one had explained "Peritoneal Dialysis" to me, so, I asked for copies of all handouts and available literature so I could spend my time in the hospital productively. The following is what I learned.

There are three types of Peritoneal Dialysis:

1. Continuous Ambulatory Peritoneal Dialysis (CAPD) the most common type. No machine is needed and it can be performed anywhere as long as its clean and adequately lit. This method occurs continuously as you walk, sit, stand, work, or play.

2. Continuous Cycling Peritoneal Dialysis (CCPD) with this type of dialysis you are connected to a machine which fills and drains the dialysate from your abdomen at night while you sleep.

3. Intermittent Peritoneal Dialysis (IPD) which uses the same type of machine and can be done at home. Usually its done in a hospital or dialysis clinic and it takes longer than (CCPD).

I chose CAPD as my method of dialysis. *See Appendix (D) for further information.*

The next visit I received was from the surgeon himself, whose purpose was to inspect my access exit site. It took no small degree of courage to look at my abdomen, which had collected as many scars as a veteran of three wars. I finally looked and discovered that I had acquired another scar and a hole on the left side of my abdomen just below the waist. From this hole hung my peritoneal dialysis access, with a square blue snap and a control with a tiny wheel which I later found out controlled the rate of flow. This access extended to the middle of my thigh. The first thought that entered my head was, "I was sure that I was one female who did not have penis envy."

We continued with my hemodialysis treatments while we waited for the peritoneal dialysis access to heal. The normal waiting period before use of this type of access is five days. Dr. Thornton was anxious to send me home so he decided to test my access in three days.

When the third day arrived, my abdominal cavity was filled with 1000 ml of dialysate. The dialysate coupled with the CO_2 which remained after surgery, produced excruciating pain. I felt an enormous amount of pressure pushing from inside-out. The gas produced so much pain in my shoulders that walking upright was difficult. When the dialysate was drained, there was a substantial amount of blood and fibrin present. I was assured that this was normal. For this purpose 1.0 cc of Heparin$^®$ was injected directly into the bags of dialysate to alleviate my fibrin problem.

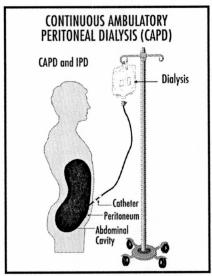

CONTINUOUS AMBULATORY PERITONEAL DIALYSIS (CAPD)

CAPD and IPD

Dialysis

Catheter
Peritoneum
Abdominal Cavity

The following day after my release from the hospital, I began my training on the proper technique to be used when doing my peritoneal dialysis treatments. I was handed a sheet of paper and asked to review the twenty-two steps included in the process. After reading through the steps several times, I was familiar enough with the theory portion of my training and ready to proceed with the practical portion, performing actual exchanges. My training continued for a period of five days. Once I felt that I was sufficiently trained, my supplies were delivered to my apartment and I was on my own.

Forty-two boxes of dialysate were stored in my bedroom which gave the impression that two of my bedroom walls were wallpapered with cardboard. My supplies included 1.5%, 2.5% and 4.5% Dextrose bags of dialysate, along with boxes of C.A.P.D. Safe-Lock® tubing, a scale, a pole to hang my dialysate bags, an Automatic Inflation Blood Pressure Monitor, syringes, Heparin®, alcohol swabs, 2 x 2 inch dressing squares, Betadyne®, and Hydrogen Peroxide®.

Supplies had to be stored at room temperature and kept away from extreme heat or cold. I was to report to the CAPD Center once every month for monitoring of my blood pressure, weight, temperature, review of medicines, drawing of blood, and discussion of my logs. These logs listed time of exchanges, percentage of dextrose in dialysate, and milliliters of dialysate used, total amount of fluid output, blood pressure, and total amount of milliliters of water removed during dialysis. I would see the nephrologist on call every month and I would have my tubing changed by a nurse. I was also provided with daytime and after hours phone numbers in case of emergencies.

It takes two to three weeks for an access site to heal. However, mine only partially healed, and the tubing moved constantly with my every action. Personal hygiene was stressed to prevent peritonitis and access site infection. I was cautioned against lifting or pulling objects weighing more than 10 pounds. Wearing loose clothes was advised to avoid irritating the access site.

The final piece of information I received concerned the first signs of peritonitis, which are: cloudy fluid being drained from the peritoneal cavity, fever, chills, headache, nausea, vomiting and moderate to severe cramps and pain in the peritoneal cavity. It took me about four weeks to become accustomed to the 1000 ml of dialysate in my peritoneal cavity. I could hear myself slosh as I walked. Sometimes I felt as though I was getting seasick from the inside out. The phrase "...and it shook when he laughed like a bowl full of jelly" took on new meaning for me. A few days later I finally overcame the queasiness I experienced while draining and filling my peritoneal cavity. Although I was told my abdomen would not become distended, it did in fact distend and I felt and looked quite pregnant.

I also felt full at all times and could eat very little, and sometimes just the thought of food made me nauseous. I was surprised at my ability to survive on the minute amount of food I was consuming. The intense gas pains continued. The pain began at my shoulders and ended at my pubic area. I also experienced irritable bowel, diarrhea and severe cramps which caused me to walk in a bent position. I discovered also that while draining or filling I frequently felt an urgent need to defecate. I felt as though I would never get accustomed to PD because the draining and filling process was very uncomfortable.

To my surprise, three months later I felt great and I was able to return to work. I was lucky to have a room with a computer available for me to continue working as I dialyzed. I could also eat an entire meal consisting of practically anything I wanted. My energy level was far superior to that experienced while on hemodialysis. PD was such a slow, gradual process that I constantly felt as though I had literally put a tiger in my tank. I might add that once my hemodialysis treatments were discontinued my anxiety attacks disappeared.

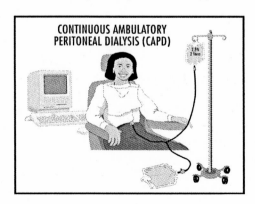

CONTINUOUS AMBULATORY
PERITONEAL DIALYSIS (CAPD)

I was asked to identify the specific food items which caused me to suffer with gas, by eliminating one food at a time and noting whether or not my symptoms were reduced. The following is a list of foods which may be gas-forming:

* Dried peas, beans, baked beans, soybeans, lima beans, and lentils.
* Cabbage, radishes, onions, broccoli, Brussels sprouts, cauliflower, and cucumbers.
* Prunes, apples, raisins, and bananas.
* Whole wheat bread, bran cereals, bran muffins.
* Milk, ice cream, ice milk and cream.
* Artificial sweeteners, high fat foods, whipped foods, and carbonated beverages.

To minimize swallowing air, I was advised to avoid: frequent, repetitive swallowing which may be caused by ill-fitting dentures, chewing gum or tobacco, sucking on hard candy or drinking beverages with a straw. Finally, the gas was alleviated with the use of Phazyme®. I avoided fried and spicy foods and consumed only bland foods to minimize the irritable bowel symptoms. After several days, I could finally walk upright and enjoyed a certain level of comfort. It was a great relief to not walk around looking like the Hunchback of Notre Dame. Also, I could actually eat, although still in very small quantities.

I did, however, experience peritonitis several times, as many peritoneal dialysis patients do. I was treated with Vancomycin. Also, using 4.25% dextrose bags of Impersol® promoted a higher propensity to contract peritonitis. I myself was required to wear a mask while hooking-up for PD, because even my own breath could enter my access and cause an infection. I also needed to keep my access exit site clean and dressed. I found that using the 2 x 2 inch sized gauze dressings with the notch was the most comfortable way to dress my access site. To allow for comfort, I began doubling my PD access in half and placing it in a baby's sized sock. My very first sock was white. It was a gift from my peritoneal dialysis nurse. My sock collection grew to the extent that I had one to match every outfit.

On one of my visits to Dr. Thornton, I complained that I had been experiencing several bouts of giant urticaria (a vascular reaction of the skin characterized by the eruption of pale evanescent wheals, associated with severe itching) and at other times a very fine rash. He said he felt it was time to increase my treatments from three to four per day and I was to increase the amount of dialysate from 1000 ml to 1500 ml. He felt that my peritoneal cavity had stretched sufficiently to accommodate the extra 500 ml of dialysate. The thought of increasing the fluid made me gag. During this time Joanne was still with me, so for her benefit we did as much sightseeing as our present conditions would allow.

As part of our recovery process we took long, slow walks on the beach which we found to be immensely therapeutic. Walking on the beach reminded us of our native island.

I was placed on a new program instituted at the Dialysis Center. When my hematocrit achieved a level of 40 gm./100 ml, my Epogen® injections were automatically discontinued. When my hematocrit level fell below 36 the injections would be initiated again. I mistakenly believed that the Epogen® injections were not required because my hematocrit was normal. In fact, Medicare only covered the cost of Epogen® injections when my hematocrit level achieved 36 gm./100 ml or below.

CHAPTER SIXTEEN

LOSS OF MY SISTER'S KIDNEY DIAGNOSED

I think that I should have no other mortal wants,
if I could always have plenty of music. It seems to infuse strength
into my limbs and ideas into my brain. Life seems to go
on without effort, when I am filled with music.

-**George Eliot**

My mental and emotional well-being by now had increased immeasurably because my energy level had increased and I had returned to work. Working had the greatest impact on my psyche. It felt as though I was a normal person leading a normal life.

On my following visit to Dr. Thornton's office, I asked him to address my hypercoagulable (excessive propensity to clot) state. I asked if there were any specific tests which would either confirm or deny the possibility that I have a coagulation (blood clotting) problem. The tests included in the coagulation panel were: PT, PTT, Bleeding time and Platelet count. The results were noncontributory except for the presence of an antiphospholipid antibody (APA) with a titer (standard of strength per volume of volumetric test solution) of 1:32. My health care team believed that finally, they had found the cause of the loss of my first transplanted kidney; that being the APA. So rare is the APA, that neither my physicians nor myself knew much about the APA except to say that it is associated with a clotting disorder.

The APA is also known as the anti-cardiolipin antibody, and was discovered in 1906. It is associated with strokes, blood clots, and decreased platelets. It is treated with anticoagulants.

It had been eight months since I had been re-activated on the kidney transplant list, and I was still working on a part-time basis. I was doing a less stressful job than before. PD was working very well and I soon returned to work full-time. I took very few bathroom breaks on PD because in a twenty-four hour period I only felt the necessity to urinate once or twice. I felt these were wasted trips because I only urinated approximately two drops.

While at work one morning, I received a telephone call at 10 a.m., from the Kidney Transplant Center with the offer of a kidney. "How was my health," asked the transplant coordinator. "Fine," I said stunned, as I sat down and digested this information. I accepted the offer and was told to proceed directly to the hospital for crossmatching, the results of which would not be available until 9 p.m. I was advised to have everything in readiness, not to have anything to eat or drink after midnght, and to await the transplant coordinator's telephone call with the test results. I turned away from the phone and with a sense of calm I announced to my co-workers that I had an offer of a kidney and needed to proceed immediately to the hospital for crossmatching.

My co-workers were all much more excited than I was and they showered me with hugs, kisses, and well wishes. They could not understand why I was not jumping for joy. I replied with the same sense of calm that there was a chance that I would not be the lucky recipient of the kidney. For that reason, I did not want to get too excited in case the crossmatch was positive. I said I would get excited when I was being wheeled into the OR.

I drove to the hospital to have the 10 to 12 tubes of blood drawn for the final crossmatching and pre-surgical workup. On returning home, I telephoned my friend Chad, a personal friend and kidney patient, to share my news. I found out that he and one other patient had also been offered the same kidney. The three of us were competing for the same kidney and being crossmatched at the same time. What would be the odds that I would be competing with a personal friend for the same kidney. I felt horrible, competing against a friend, especially one whose need for a kidney transplant was indeed greater than my own. I secretly prayed that I would not be the recipient of the kidney and that Chad would be.

While I waited for the test results, I packed my bag, cleaned my apartment, dumped the trash, did the wash, cleaned the refrigerator, paid all bills, and changed the bedclothes.

Fanny was again given the keys to my apartment and mailbox. My friend Suzanne offered to take care of Jake my cockatiel, and Sarah waited with me for the telephone call so she could rush me to the hospital if the need arose.

It was 9:15 p.m., when the call finally came through. John the transplant coordinator said he had bad news, "You did not get the kidney." I then asked if he could tell me if Chad was the recipient, he said, "No, it went to another patient."

I felt a wave of sadness wash over me, not for myself, but for Chad. This was my first offer of a kidney but Chad had experienced this several times before. I could not imagine how he felt. A few days later he admitted to me that he was angry. He was getting tired of waiting.

CHAPTER SEVENTEEN

MY SISTER RETURNS HOME

> *One of the things I learned the hard way was that it doesn't pay to get discouraged. Keeping busy and making optimism a way of life can restore your faith in yourself.*
>
> **-Lucille Ball**

Joanne was seriously considering relocating to the States. Although she would enjoy being with me, she would miss the island, our father, and her circle of friends too much to stay. In short, she had an established life on the island that she wished to return to. Her decision to return home was precipitated by the fact that I was back on my feet physically and emotionally. Although I understood her need to return to the Caribbean, I could not help but experience a sense of disappointment, because it had been 20 years since we both lived in the same country. In the six months that she spent with me, I had grown accustomed to having her around.

I now had the unhappy task of setting the date for her departure and purchasing her airline ticket. I asked Chad to drive us to the airport because I knew that I would be too emotional.

Too soon the day I dreaded arrived. Chad arrived early. He drove slowly to the airport to allow Joanne ample time for a last look around before she left. We arrived at the airport, Joanne checked-in, and I sat stiff-lipped fighting back the tears at the thought of saying good-bye to my sister.

Finally, the departure of Joanne's flight was announced and instantly both Joanne and I burst into tears. We clung to each other and could not let go until Chad was obliged to pry us apart, so he could say his good-bye and Joanne could board the airplane. I was engulfed by an intense wave of sadness because I knew my apartment would seem empty without her. I was inconsolable. Chad did not know what he could do to comfort me. I believe he took me with him as he accomplished his chores because he knew that if left alone I would be depressed and probably spend the rest of the day crying.

Four months after Joanne's departure, I had adjusted to being alone again. I was watching television around 3:30 p.m., and had just dropped off to sleep when the phone rang. It was John, the transplant coordinator, asking if I still had an interest in transplantation. When I said of course, he told me that the kidney was being flown in from the midwest and would arrive at St. Michael's Hospital at 9 p.m.

John also said that Chad and I were the only two patients competing for the kidney. Chad did have first option should both our crossmatch results be negative, because he has been on the transplant list for a longer period of time. If Chad was not able to accept the kidney because of a positive crossmatch, illness, surgery, or infection, I would be the alternate recipient.

As before, I reported to the laboratory at St. Michael's hospital for testing, made the usual preparations and waited for the results. I received the telephone call at 4 a.m., and I heard the familiar words, "I have bad news. I am sorry to say that you did not get the kidney, maybe next time." The first time I heard these words it took me twenty-four hours to deal with the disappointment. This time I was half asleep when I received the telephone call. After I hung up the phone, I went back to sleep until my clock alarm rang and woke me at my regularly appointed time 5:45 a.m. The following morning my co-workers were all shocked to see me. They were disappointed that I was not the kidney recipient. Chad did not receive the kidney either. The kidney had to be sent to another transplant facility where there were other hopeful recipients.

While watching television the following evening I was suddenly gripped by a wave of sadness, almost depression. It took me a few minutes to realize why I felt so badly. I was having a delayed reaction to the fact that I was not the recipient of the kidney.

As I waited for my kidney over the following year and a half, I would suffer many bouts of peritonitis. I experienced a particularly bad infection on Halloween at 2 a.m. Wearing my robe and slippers, I drove myself to the hospital doubled over in pain while maintaining a death grip on the steering wheel of my car. I was forced to take shallow, rapid breaths to minimize the pain, and it was not until I received an injection of Demerol® at the hospital that my pain began to subside.

Dialyzing in the hospital was a frustrating experience. The nurses insisted on performing the dialysis for me. Most of the nurses had never actually dialyzed a patient before and the only one who had, had not done so in many years, and had to rely on outdated instructions for the outdated equipment. For all these reasons, the process which should have taken half an hour took at least one and a half hours.

It was determined that I had a staphylococcus epidermidis infection which required the use of antibiotics. Once the antibiotics were initiated, I was released from the hospital.

On my follow-up visit to Dr. Thornton, he shared with me that he felt I should remove my name from the Kidney Transplant List for a year, and give serious

73

thought to how aggressively I wanted to pursue transplantation. His rationale being that I was doing very well on peritoneal dialysis and taking relatively very few medications. He also said that he would hate to see me trading something that works well, for something I believed to be better, and realize too late that transplantation was not really a good option for me.

He further explained that the patient he saw before me was having a difficult time with a thrush/yeast infection in his mouth and throat. The infection had become so unbearably problematic that he begged Dr. Thornton to help alleviate his symptoms because he could no longer endure it.

Dr. Thornton responded by saying he could not prescribe the antifungals required to control the infection without the risk of killing his transplanted kidney. The only other option available was to discontinue the immunosuppressants, but this would ultimately result in the loss of his transplanted kidney, and his return to hemodialysis. The patient then said that he would not return to hemodialysis, and would resign himself to living with the discomfort. Dr. Thornton said that he would hate to see me suffering the same fate. I have to admit that the idea of staying on peritoneal dialysis had occurred to me. I had heard the horror stories about the complications resulting from the use of the potent anti-rejection medications all transplant patients are required to take. This idea gave me pause.

I discussed the possibility of not having the second transplant with other kidney transplant patients and their responses were the same. "You just think you feel well right now. You don't remember how it is to feel truly well. You've accepted feeling badly and tired for so long that it has become a normal way of life. After transplantation, you feel as you did before you got sick. You've got to have the transplant." I was now provided with more food for thought. What a dilemma. I approached this life-altering decision very cautiously for fear of making a mistake.

The waiting continued. Every time a pocket pager beeped in my vicinity my heart did a somersault and my stomach became a clenched fist. Most of the pages were not legitimate, and you only learned this by responding to the pages.

Dr. Thornton left the medical facility where I was being treated. I was forced to continue my follow-up care with another nephrologist. I had grown accustomed to Dr. Thornton in the five years I had been his patient, and I hated the thought of starting over with another nephrologist.

CHAPTER EIGHTEEN

THE FREEDOM CYCLER®

> *Illness is the doctor to whom we pay most heed;*
> *to kindness, to knowledge, we make promises only;*
> *pain we obey.*
>
> **-Marcel Proust**

On my first appointment with the new nephrologist, Dr. Peter VanWagenen, I mentioned that I was concerned about my weight gain. He asked how many cycles I performed a day and what were the concentrations of dextrose in the bags of dialysate I was using. After I responded, he said that he was not surprised that I was experiencing a weight gain, because of the concentrations of the bags of dialysate I was using, I was consuming between 1200-1500 calories a day in dialysate alone without taking a single bite of food.

He changed my prescription, asking me to cycle five instead of four times a day, and use two 1.5% dextrose bags and three 2.5% dextrose bags of dialysate. He advised me to avoid the use of the 4.25% dextrose bags of dialysate as much as possible since this higher concentration could, over time, destroy the effectiveness of my peritoneum.

After implementing the change in prescription, my laboratory results revealed that my creatinine had lowered from 14.6 to 12.0 mg/dL and my BUN went from 80 to 50 mg/dL. I did feel a little better and had more energy, which Dr. Vanwagenen said was purely coincidental. I had been told in the past that in one experiment, while on dialysis, patients were injected with creatinine. The result was that the patient's creatinine values were the same at the end of their dialysis sessions as when they began. The patients still felt better after their dialysis session even though their creatinine levels remained the same.

I could always tell when my creatinine and BUN levels were very high because I would experience the same unpleasant taste and odor in my mouth. I also experienced aching joints and muscle spasms all over my body especially in my face and neck. These symptoms could also be produced by low electrolytic levels. For this reason I always kept a supply of Gatorade® or Powerade® in my refrigerator, especially in the summertime.

To eliminate these problems, I began brushing my teeth several times a day and always kept Clorets® gum on hand. Once the values were lowered the odor would no longer be problematic. I chewed such a quantity of Clorets® gum that I probably singlehandedly boosted the value of their stock on the exchange.

My five cycles a day fit into my daily schedule very easily. The first I performed while blowdrying my hair and applying my makeup. The second cycle during my mid morning break at work, the third cycle during my mid afternoon break, the fourth cycle during dinner, and the fifth cycle while reading, before I went to sleep at night.

My luck continued running true to form. The new nephrologist resigned. This time I was told that my followup appointment would be with yet another nephrologist. To say that I was not ecstatic with the news would be putting it mildly.

Once I find a physician who provides me with excellent medical care, and with whom I achieve a certain comfort level and rapport, it is very traumatic to have to see someone else. For me, the trauma and stress was heightened because of my life threatening disease. I see my health care professionals as my lifeline. Losing a physician I trust, is akin to losing my lifeline.

Dr. Harry Lee, the new nephrologist was quiet, thorough, concerned, and possessed a very dry sense of humor. He also did not laugh very much. I told him that I was not having much success with my weight loss program. The additional weight was causing my ankles, knees, and back to ache. He ordered a Peritoneal Equilibrium Test (PET) to check the level of function of my peritoneal membrane.

He also ordered a Kinetics X Volume/Urea (KT/V) test to check for adequate dialysis and creatinine clearance. Based on the results, he deduced that I was not being adequately dialyzed and my body was absorbing all the sugar/dextrose from the dialysate. He recommended I use the Freedom Cycler® (peritoneal dialysis machine) at nights while I slept. This would provide adequate dialysis which would take place at a more rapid rate, preventing my body from absorbing all the dextrose in the dialysate. Dr. Lee also recommended the addition of Vitamin E to my medications. Vitamin E is believed to lower the incidence of heart disease which dialysis patients are very prone to developing.

The dextrose content in the dialysate elevated my cholesterol and triglycerides levels. They were both between 500-700 mg/dL (normal less than 229 mg/dL and 122 mg/dL respectively), which is high even for a peritoneal dialysis patient. Lipitor® was added to my medications to lower these values. Next, came my training on the Freedom Cycler®.

The Freedom Cycler® is not big or heavy, but cumbersome. It has the appearance of a box about 15 x 10 x 12 inches in maximum dimensions and is mounted on a pole, which has four legs extending out from the pole at its base. Although equipped with wheels, it does not move easily on carpet.

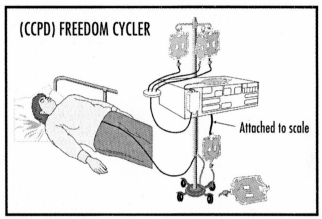

(CCPD) FREEDOM CYCLER

Attached to scale

The face of the machine is equipped with a display which gives several readings: # exchanges, fill volume, last fill, fill time, dwell time, drain time, time left, options, data sheet (running total of amount of fluid filled and drained), clock, and start and stop buttons. The face also has a select button, up and down arrows for moving up and down within the menu and data sheet. Once my training was completed, I was given my cycler to take home. I had difficulty assembling the Freedom Cycler® so I enlisted the help of my dear friend David Anthony.

For the first two weeks, I experienced multiple problems with the cycler. Once I was hooked-up to the cycler it did not allow me the freedom to reach the refrigerator, get a drink or reach the bathroom to urinate.

One morning around 2 a.m., I found myself dragging the cycler as far as it would go, then stretched the tubing tethering me to the cycler to half its normal size in an attempt to reach the commode. If you could detach and reattach yourself to the cycler numerous times, I would not have had to execute such an elaborate ballet in an attempt to accomplish what otherwise are considered normal activities of living.

On another occasion, I detached myself from the cycler so I could use the bathroom and had to replace the Y-set tubing. This takes some time to do especially at 2 a.m. when you are half asleep. Once the tubing was replaced and I was tethered to the cycler again, it took quite a while to fall asleep again. Two weeks of this resulted in my becoming sleep deprived, edgy, and irritable. Because I was in a constant state of listlessness and exhaustion, it was a huge struggle for me to use the Freedom Cycler®. For example, I had difficulty lifting the two 5000 ml bags of dialysate and loading them on the tray on top of the cycler.

Once the drain bags which hung from below the cycler were filled and in need of disposal, it required a huge effort to lift the bags for draining. It became my practice to drag them across the carpet into the bathroom then lift and maneuver the bags into the bathtub. The final step was to cut the bags, disposing of the waste fluid. I wondered how older or more feeble patients were managing if I was having such a struggle?

The alarm problem grew worse as the days flew by and the nights seemed endless. The alarm sounded so many times during the night that it threw me completely off my schedule. By the time my clock alarm rang heralding my time to get out of bed, I would be one or two cycles short of my total daily requirement of five cycles.

I was not being adequately dialyzed and I knew that the impurities were increasing in my blood stream because I felt badly. The way I felt was always my best indication of how well I was doing healthwise. Usually, I could tell which value was out of range by the specific symptoms I was experiencing. For example, a low calcium would produce achy bones and muscle spasms in my feet and legs, while a high potassium produced nausea and vomiting, and diarrhea.

Everything became an effort. My legs felt as though they weighed one hundred pounds each, I experienced lightheadedness sporadically, and there was a constant feeling of exhaustion. I noticed that my fingers and toes began to feel numb and my tongue and legs experienced a tingling sensation.

The following day my hands, feet and tongue felt almost completely numb. I also felt as though I was on the verge of fainting. When I began having a problem holding my head erect I panicked and asked my friend David Anthony to take me to the emergency room at St. Ignatius hospital.

As soon as I arrived at the ER, blood was drawn and sent to the laboratory for testing on a STAT basis. When the results were received I was told that my potassium was 7.5 mEq/L and my BUN was 98 mg/dL. "You are seriously underdialyzed," said the emergency room physician. I was not admitted to the hospital, but instead I was given Compazine® for the nausea and Kayexalate® to drink which produced diarrhea. This is the easiest way to remove excess potassium from the body. I was directed to increase my cycles to six or seven each day in order to reduce the level of impurities or toxins in my system.

The nurse was shocked. She said, "We never send patients home with laboratory values as high as yours, but since it is you, the doctor said that you can be trusted to be compliant, so we are sending you home." It took several days before the numbness and tingling wore off and I was able to return to work.

The Freedom Cycler® was supposed to be more efficient, increase the quality of my dialysis treatments, and afford me a greater degree of freedom during the day. The cycler did in fact allow me greater freedom during the day but limited my freedom at night by requiring that I be home at an early hour. My CAPD or manual dialysis in fact fit perfectly into my work and activities schedules.

I had to be tethered to the cycler by a certain hour in order to obtain the required amount of treatments before my appointed time to awaken in the morning. In other words, if I did anything on a week night and did not return home by a certain hour I would be short at least one treatment or one cycle. With CAPD, my cycles were timed so I only had one cycle left to perform before I went to bed at night.

Traveling was much easier with a few boxes of dialysate and Y-sets rather than having to carry the cycler as well. The cycler could not be used on any moving mode of conveyance, such as cars, boats, planes, and trains. The motion would set off the alarm and have to be reset each time the alarm sounded.

While this method did not work for me, my friend, Douglas, however, who is thriving with the use of the Freedom Cycler®. Douglas is therefore, a strong advocate of this method of PD. This is yet another prime example of all things not working for all people. It is essential to carefully select the method that suits your lifestyle while providing adequate dialysis.

CHAPTER NINETEEN

MY SECOND KIDNEY TRANSPLANT

You gain strength, courage and confidence by every
experience in which you really stop to look fear in the face....
You must do the thing you cannot do.

-Eleanor Roosevelt

At the 10:40 p.m., showing of Jurassic Park The Lost World, with two of my friends, my pocket pager beeped and sent me rushing to the foyer to respond to the page. I saw several police officers standing in conversation and asked them for the location of the payphones. One of the officers indicated the payphones as I reached into my fanny pack to find a quarter, and realized to my horror that I only had dollar bills. I quickly explained my situation and the officer reached into his pocket and retrieved a handful of coins, selected a quarter and handed it to me and said, "Here's a quarter, good luck." I gratefully accepted the quarter, thanked him profusely, and ran toward the payphones. I placed the call and waited for a response from the Transplant Center answering service. Finally, the response came, I had not been beeped.

In that moment, I told myself that I had false alarms before and I was sure there would be false alarms in my future. Therefore, there was no point of allowing myself to become upset, otherwise by the time I actually got my kidney I would be a "basket case."

At this point in my illness I had already experienced the anger, depression, acceptance, and finally the change of attitude phases of the process. This is a process which all patient's with life threatening diseases inevitably experience. It was not anyone's fault that I had a hereditary disease. There was also no point to becoming angry or depressed over a situation that was completely out of my control.

By the end of the movie, the amount of fluid in my peritoneal cavity was so great that I was uncomfortable and had difficulty breathing. I went to the restroom to drain some of the fluid. I was standing facing the commode when another cinema patron entered the adjacent stall. It occurred to me that the person next door might notice the direction of my feet and the fact that I was standing facing the fixture and "going" for what seemed a very long time. I was reluctant to leave the stall and decided to wait until the person next door had left the restroom. Had I been the cinema patron in the adjacent stall, I know my curiosity would have been aroused. Had the patron actually seen me, I imagined her speculating as to whether or not I was a transvestite, and marveling at what a remarkable job the plastic surgeon had done. I have to admit that I felt silly for even considering such a thought.

While my waiting on the transplant list continued, I occupied my time by cleaning out my closets, keeping in touch with old friends and family, had my will redrawn, and generally put my house in order. I also began investigating Advance Medical Directives which can take the form of a Living Will or Durable Power of Attorney. *See Appendix (E) for further information.*

Although I managed to occupy my time, my patience was beginning to wear thin. At the present time I knew that I was healthier than I had been in the last six years and all my instincts were telling me that I was ready. I waited two and a half years for my kidney transplant which is not a long time to wait considering many patients wait for much longer periods of time. The sixth time was the charm for me. I guess walking around my apartment singing "All I Want for Christmas Is A New Kidney, A New Kidney, A New Kidney..." really did work.

I will never forget the day I got the telephone call with the offer of "the kidney." It was December 19th at approximately noon and I was at work. I left work shortly thereafter to have my crossmatching performed at St. Michael's Hospital. At approximately 11:30 p.m., I was awakened by the sound of the telephone ringing. It was John, the transplant coordinator, with the news that the kidney was a three antigen match and that the final crossmatch was negative.

I accepted the offer of the kidney and was told to report to St. Michael's Hospital at 7 a.m., the following morning, December 20th, for transplantation. What an unbelievable Christmas present. My bag had been packed and waiting for a very long time. I had only to throw my toiletries into the bag, call Sarah, who was on permanent alert for my ride to the hospital, and give David Anthony the key to my apartment so he could care for Jake.

Dr. Garcia, the anesthesiologist and the rest of the surgical team were already present when we arrived. I was immediately prepared for surgery, this time Dilaudid®, not Morphine® was administered and I was taken to the OR. Dr. Taber said that all of my blood samples for the year were crossmatched with the donor, and all but one sample reacted negatively. The positive sample was taken shortly after I had experienced a cold. Also, several consultations took place with nephrologists, and hematologists from two medical facilities during the twenty-four hours prior to my transplant. The consultations were to determine what level of anticoagulation should be used both during and post transplantation. Extreme care was being taken because of the loss of my previous allograft and because I still tested positively for the antiphospholipid antibody. This set a new precedent for transplant surgery for all transplant patients with an antiphospholipid antibody who would follow in my footsteps at the Transplant Center.

I must confess to a certain apprehension before my second transplant, because I had learned from prior experience that complications can occur. This time, however, everything went well, and I felt terrific the following day. My two-day stay in the hospital was remarkably pain free, then I was released into the care of my loving boyfriend David Anthony. Within eight hours the Dilaudid® wore off and the overwhelming pain set in. Again, Percocet® was there to provide me with pain relief, enhancing my comfort level.

My list of post transplant medications included: Neoral®, (new form of cyclosporin), Cellcept®, Prednisone®, Zantac® (ranitidine), Dipyridamole®, Bactrim DS® (SMZ-TMS DS), Nystatin®, Amphogel®, Nu-Iron®, Cytovene® (ganciclovir), Lasix® (furosemide), Coumadin®, Neutra-Phos®, Phenergan® (promethazine), Ambien®, Xanax® (alprazolam), Percocet® (roxicet), and Lipitor® (atrorastatin).

The Neoral® was my least favorite medication to take because of its pungent odor which caused me to be nauseous. I invested in an immense pill box which held two weeks worth of all my medications. This kept me from missing doses of my medication and at the same time aired the Neoral® making the odor less offensive and the capsules easier to swallow without experiencing nausea.

A patient who does not take his/her medications as prescribed is considered noncompliant. Noncompliance is the third most common cause of transplant failure. It was explained to me that under extenuating circumstances if one dose of my medications was missed, it was not critical. However, I should never, under any circumstances, miss two consecutive doses because this could precipitate a rejection episode. I was also cautioned against discontinuing or making changes to my medication dosages unless specifically directed to do so by my transplant coordinator.

Being the cautious person that I am, I took this one step further. Before taking any medications e.g., medications to treat a cough, cold, or allergies, I always checked with my transplant coordinator to be sure that I would not experience an anaphylactic reaction (a hypersensitive state or acute reaction brought about by allergic reaction to a medication or incompatibility between medications) with any of the medications I was already taking.

I was given a chart to keep a record of my medication intake and to refer to for proper dosing. These charts were in a manila folder which I will take with me to each visit with my transplant coordinator so he/she can make changes in dosages as required. If I throw up or miss a dose of medications, I was advised to call my Transplant Coordinator for instructions.

I was told that I would experience numerous side effects during the first year post transplantation while the initial dosage of my medications are high. I was encouraged to be tough, and be aware that these side effects are temporary and know that I was going to make it. I was cautioned against vaccination and Flu-shots because it is believed that they are not effective for the first two years post transplantation.

With all this information, I felt as though I was forewarned, therefore, fore-armed. I resolved not to worry, and looked forward to my transplant with wild anticipation and excitement.

CHAPTER TWENTY

ADJUSTING TO
POST TRANSPLANT MEDICATIONS

> *If we let things terrify us, life will not be worth living.*
> **-Seneca, Epistles**

After transplantation, I was advised to resume my normal daily activities because I was no longer viewed as a sick patient but as a normal, healthy recipient. I was provided a list of recommendations to follow to protect my new kidney.

* Get a doctor's release before returning to work or school.
* No contact sports.
* If I plan to travel carry medicines with me and not in my
 luggage in case of loss.
* Carry an ID card identifying myself as a transplant recipient.
* Know the location of the Transplant Center closest to my
 destination.
* Sexual relations may be resumed four to six weeks post transplantation
 or when I feel up to the task. *See Appendix (F) for more detailed
 information.*

Other instructions included: calling my transplant coordinator immediately in case of fever. Never wait until Friday evening or during the weekend to call if I have been feeling badly for more than two days. It may be difficult to contact a physician during that time. Do not call the transplant coordinator at home or on the weekends with questions that should be dealt with during office visits, e.g., diet, exercise or prescription refills.

Inevitably I would forget to ask a question or mention a new symptom, therefore, I made lists to take with me to my office visits. I also kept track of my prescriptions and phoned in my refill orders "before" I ran out of my medications.

Due to the high doses of immunosuppressants/steroids for the following four weeks, I existed in an alternate drug induced world. In this world I felt as though I was evolving into someone else. I was unable to control my emotions, mood swings or changes in my personality. My fingers and toes burned unbearably as though on fire and I was experiencing nightmares of such horrific proportions that I could not bring myself to recount them. I felt as though I was the bride of Frankenstein or a medical experiment gone awry. Then I began experiencing anxiety, sleeplessness, bloating, frequent urination (a new experience), extreme hunger and headaches.

On my follow-up visit with Dr. Taber, I discussed my list of symptoms. Our discussion resulted in a decrease in the dosage of the Neoral® to eliminate the nightmares and the Prednisone® to decrease the burning in my fingers and toes and my mood swings. I was prescribed Xanax ® for my anxiety and Ambien® to sleep at night.

During the fifth week of my recovery, I was able to discontinue the Percocet® for pain control and take it on a PRN (as needed) basis only. The next symptom I experienced was excruciating, stabbing and throbbing pain in my lower extremities. I could barely move let alone walk. This was the result of a very low phosphorous level. To alleviate this problem my Neutra-Phos® was increased along with my intake of phosphorous-rich foods, the same foods I was obliged to avoid during dialysis. It did take, however, 48 hours before the Neutra-Phos® and phosphorous-rich foods would take effect. I turned once again to Percocet® for pain relief.

The mood and personality alteration symptoms persisted. I was assured that this is normal and that my case was mild. Some patients experience drug-induced behavior which borders on the psychotic. They exhibit violent behavior to the point of throwing chairs through their windows and smashing their television sets. I also became short tempered and easily irritated by the most minute of issues. One minute I experienced extreme anger, the next, I would lapse into depression and burst into tears. Luckily, I was not at work, but at home alone recuperating during this trying period.   My symptoms were discussed with my transplant coordinator, which again resulted in the decrease in dosage of certain medications. I also began sleeping through the night and not staying awake for two to three consecutive days. I was beginning to feel more like myself.

I then began experiencing cravings for peanuts, bananas, grapefruit, orange and apple juices, sweets and deserts. Grapefruit, I discovered, is taboo for immunosuppressed patients. The grapefruit reacts in a certain way with the Neoral® inhibiting the action of the chemical P450. P450 promotes the passage of the Neoral® through the liver to be excreted. Without excretion, the Neoral® continues circulating within my system at a constant level, until other doses are taken. This has an accumulative effect and could increasing the Neoral® to a toxic level.

The Neoral® caused me to shake both inside and out. My stomach felt as though it was constantly quivering, and the trembling in my hands caused my handwriting to change. Applying makeup became a challenge. Applying lipstick specifically, takes me back to my childhood, when one of my greatest accomplishments was keeping my crayon within the lines of the drawing I was coloring.

Several weeks later two new symptoms made their appearance. The first was a lowering of my blood pressure to 110/60 mm/Hg coupled with lightheadedness. The second was bursting blood vessels causing extreme bruising and edema (swelling). This was the result of my being too anticoagulated and my Coumadin®, Dipyridamole® and aspirin anticoagulation medications had to be adjusted to correct the problem.

The second symptom took the form of what I call bloat. This is a combination of thickening of the underlying tissue beneath the skin and a redistribution of my body fat by the Prednisone®. Unfortunately, the bloat concentrated on my face, starting with the cheeks, eyelids and bags under the eyes, followed by the neck, shoulders, and a fat pad at the nape of my neck extending between the shoulder blades. I was told that as the dosage of Prednisone® was decreased, so too would the bloat. Realistically, I should not expect any significant improvement for at least another 9-12 months.

Approximately one month later, another symptom reared its ugly head. This time it took the form of excessive dark hair growth on my entire face, ears including the earlobes, throat, back of the neck, shoulders, down the center of my back and my arms. I was obliged to initiate the use of a hair removal system once a week. This new ritual I referred to as "defurring myself." Consequently, when anyone asked me how I was doing, I would respond that I was constantly trying to keep from changing into a male or a shaggy dog. Even worse, I could be changing into a male dog, so in the event I was observed lifting my leg in an attempt to mark my territory, they should stop me before I did anything to embarrass myself.

David Anthony with his unique sense of humor told me one night while I was complaining about the excessive hair grown, "Honey, I've been meaning to tell you I think you're more man than I can handle," not to be outdone, in jest I responded, "I know, why just this morning I caught myself scratching my crotch and spitting."

Several weeks later, I began experiencing symptoms similar to a bladder infection: pressure on the bladder, painful urination, and frequency of urination every 5-10 minutes. I was also experiencing a certain amount of aching from my allograft. Dr. Taber ordered a Urinalysis which was negative, indicating that my problem was other than a bladder infection. He then ordered an ultrasound of the donor kidney which revealed that the donor kidney was fine.

I also had a CT scan beginning at my navel and ending at my pubic area. This revealed a large lymphocele (a sac or pocket containing a collection of fluid) which was applying pressure on both my donor kidney and bladder, and would require surgery in order to drain. One hour later, I was in surgery having 300 ccs of fluid drained from the lymphocele.

At two months post transplantation I began feeling a little more like the Donna of old. I was still very cautious, however, about making any major decisions which would affect the rest of my life. I recognized that it would be some time before I would feel one hundred percent physically and emotionally, because the dosages of my medications were still relatively high. At this time I was still given to bouts of anger, depression and crying although not as severe as before.

I continued to occupy my time with daily walks, cross-word puzzles, reading books and magazines and watching a brain-numbing amount of television. I also listened to my favorite music which always seemed to have a soothing effect. I set goals regarding my recovery, diet, and exercise regimen and yet other future goals to be accomplished once I was fully recovered. This imprinted on my psyche a sense of continuity, that I had a future, and was going to survive.

At my worst point emotionally, I actually sat down with pen and paper and made a list of everything I could think of that I should be grateful for in my life. The list was extensive. The first item on my list was, I am alive! Somehow seeing the list in black and white impressed upon me just how lucky and privileged I was.

The time had now come to write my donor family to express my gratitude for their precious gift of a kidney. *See Appendix (G) for a list of guidelines for writing to donor families.*

To my surprise, writing my donor family was one of the most difficult tasks I had undertaken. Initially, I experienced an overwhelming sense of guilt that someone had to die so that I could have a second chance at a "normal life." I dealt with this guilt by rationalizing that I did not control the fact that I inherited a kidney disease any more than I controlled the fact that it was my donor's time to go beyond to his eternal progression.

It came as no surprise that my donor family did not respond to my letter because I never expected a response. For me, thanking my donor family was a necessary part of my recovery. I felt good about the fact that I did what I thought was the right thing to do. Some donor families take the opportunity anonymously, to express to the recipient, what a wonderful person the donor was in life. In some cases, the donor families have been known to send the recipient a photograph or a personal item of the donor along with their letter of response. In yet other instances the donor family welcomes the opportunity to meet the recipient.

Along with my frequent bladder infections I also began experiencing UTIs (urinary tract infections). Immunosuppressed females have a high incidence of asymptomatic bladder infections or UTIs such as staphylococcus and streptococcus, which are normal flora on the human skin. These infections are usually cured by the body's immune system. Because of immunosuppression my body could not accomplish this on its own. Therefore, my immune system was given help to combat the infections through the use of antibiotics, such as Bactrim®, Orfloxacin®, Cipro®, Macrodantin® or Amikacin®.

Warning signs that you may have a UTI include:

* Pain.
* Burning during urination.
* Feeling an urgent need to urinate frequently
  though the amount of urine may be small.
* Getting up often at night to pass urine.
* Cloudy, bloody or foul smelling urine.

See Appendix (H) for further information.

For me, an additional concern because of immunosuppression was the contraction of Psittacosis also knows as (parrot fever, ornithosis or chlamydiosis). Transmission occurs through contact with sick birds shedding the organisms especially when stressed. For this reason I took Jake to an avian veterinarian for testing. The trip to the veterinarian was stressful for both Jake and myself. All the trauma was worth it when a few days later I received the negative result of his Psittacosis test.

Warning signs of Psittacosis in humans include: persistent flu-like symptoms such as fever, chills, headache, weakness, fatigue and respiratory signs. If this occurs the bird must be treated by a qualified avian veterinarian and you must consult your physician immediately because these organisms could be potentially dangerous.

CHAPTER TWENTY-ONE

DIET, EXERCISE, AND HEAD-GAMES

> *Life is a warfare; and he who easily desponds deserts a*
> *double duty: he betrays the noblest property of man,*
> *which is dauntless resolution; and he rejects the providence*
> *of that all gracious Being who guides and rules the universe.*
> **-Jane Porter**

A problem shared by all transplant patients is excessive weight gain. In my case the weight gain was due to the following factors:

* Food was more enjoyable than when I was in renal failure.
* Dietary restrictions were lifted.
* I was prone to overeating.
* Prednisone® increased my appetite.
* Prednisone® caused my body to make fat and lose muscle.

Dr. Taber advised me to monitor my caloric intake. I had already accepted the fact that realistically, I could not expect any significant weight loss for at least one year. At one year post transplantation, the steroids are reduced to a level which will allow weight loss. The object is to practice good nutrition and health without excessive weight gain by restricting salt intake, and including foods from all food groups in the diet, but in moderation.

It is necessary for kidney transplant patients to eat an adequate amount of protein because the Neoral® (cyclosporin) relies on protein to react and be effective.

Weight gain can cause an alteration of appearance, hypertension, and diabetes, which could adversely affect my new kidney. Medication dosage may have to be increased because dosage of certain medications is estimated according to weight. In my case, my weight gain was estimated at twenty pounds, and my appearance and facial features were altered to the point that I saw a stranger looking back from my mirror. In my opinion, my face has aged approximately 10 years. I am still learning to love my new face.

I was admonished to always seek the help of a Dietitian when planning a diet. Custom order foods when eating out, e.g., order Chinese food without Monosodium Glutamate (MSG). Chinese food is an excellent source of vegetables and starch protein.

Exercise is just as important as taking medications and maintaining proper nutrition. The basic rules include:

* Make an exercise plan and stick to it.
* Make a commitment to good health and well-being.
* Set work-out goals and chart my progress.
* Have realistic expectations.
* Start slow with short walks.
* Avoid excessive exposure to heat.
* Limit exercise sessions to 20-30 minutes.
* Reward myself for my hard work.
* View my lapses and setbacks as challenges.
* Re-evaluate my plan and add variety as needed.
* Stop exercising if I experience tiredness, dizziness, cramps, shortness of breath or nausea.
* Do not exercise if I have pain, fever, or generally do not feel well.

Exercise can reduce stress, improve posture and sleep, and provide better digestion and could protect me against diseases. Exercise also increases my energy level and provides better emotional and psychological well-being. Most kidney patients live normal healthy lives filled with activity. Some even exceed their transplant team's expectations. For example, 2,200 transplant patients from 58 countries around the world, traveled to Sidney, Australia to compete in the XI World Transplant Games, and the number of participants continues to increase. What a coup for the participants, to have achieved such a degree of excellence in recovery and physical condition.

During stressful moments, I have always been given to having conversations with myself while looking in the mirror. I refer to this process as "head-games." Even though "head-games" have always worked for me, I was reluctant to admit that I talked to myself. I discovered that this process is a widely accepted form of therapy which is viewed as quite normal and a very useful, even powerful tool.

One head-game I played with myself is countering my negative thoughts by saying cancel, cancel, and replacing the negative thought with a positive one. I then think the positive thought at least three times to completely replace the negative with the positive. Playing positive "head-games" changed my mood, behavior and helped me maintain a positive mental attitude.

Positive "head-games" also had a direct effect on how I interpreted and dealt with my particular set of circumstances. Positive as well as negative "head-games" can both become self-fulfilling prophecy. I never lost sight of the fact that I was after rationality coupled with accuracy and not self-delusion.

Overall, I am a very positive and upbeat person who subscribes to the belief that laughter is healing and therapeutic. Actual studies have proven that laughter can sustain the immune system, whereas stress and anger do the reverse. I managed to find humor in most of my challenges. The exceptions were those few times when my situation was so grave that I became overwhelmed. These are the moments in which I prayed most fervently.

I shared the funny aspects of my challenges with family, friends, and other transplant patients. Transplant patients share a special bond brought about by the fact that we are going through the same physical, emotional and psychological changes.

Associating with transplant patients makes some recipients feel normal. This had quite the reverse effect on me and I felt better being among my so-called normal friends. Whenever possible I carried on much as I did before my disease became apparent and I became seriously ill. I was and still am determined to recapture as much as is realistically possible of the life I had prior to kidney disease. This, truly makes me feel normal. Feeling normal or good about myself is a very powerful restorative. Each individual needs to find what works for them and implement it in their daily lives.

Personally, I watched a lot of comedies, read funny books and cards, told jokes, talked cheerfully and smiled frequently. I added Erma Bombeck, Loretta LaRoche and Sarah Ban Breathnach to my reading repertoire and they soon became numbered among my favorites.

Another adjustment was not being compulsive about cleaning. It was not possible sometimes because I was weak and tired easily. I then adopted what I term the one hundred year rule, "In one hundred years is it going to matter that I did not dust or vacuum." If the answer was no, then it just did not matter. Among the other "head-games" I played with myself was listening to inspirational tapes, books on tape and my favorite music, at home and in my car. I avoided associating with people who were usually very negative. I know this seems extreme but I could not allow myself to get depressed, it took me several days to regain positive ground once I became depressed.

When talking did not have a positive effect, I wrote. As already mentioned, over the course of two and a half years while I waited for my kidney transplant, I managed to fill several writing tablets with my experiences. Here again, I was exercising what I thought to be common sense, not realizing that I was on target with widely accepted and practiced methods of therapy.

The MENTOR program also had a huge impact in my life. My mentor, Ruben Ochoa, was someone I met through the Kidney Transplant Center who was five years post kidney transplantation and a diabetic. Ruben was a great source of information answering my many questions and addressing my concerns. I was fortunate to have someone to counsel me, who had traveled the road on which I now found myself, and with whom I shared a unique fellowship. In the beginning, Ruben and I talked several times a day, any time, day or night, and our conversations were lengthy, in depth and very candid.

I could never bring myself to join a support group although I do believe they provide significant benefits. I myself, am reluctant to introduce certain intimate topics or concerns in a group setting. For this reason, I felt that my legitimate questions would go unanswered. This is one example of how the MENTOR program with its counseling on a one to one basis, has the edge. This program provides a certain comfort level which allows transplant recipients to openly discuss their concerns and have them addressed. *See Appendix (I) for further information.* Also, I am lucky to have a wide circle of friends and family members to turn to for support.

For those transplant patients who are not as fortunate, the MENTOR program can be of significant benefit. I look forward to the day when I too can become a mentor and help someone else down the road that I am now travelling.

The Transplant Recipients International Organization (TRIO) provides "Hot Line Mentors" for transplant patients and their family members. TRIO sends a letter to each candidate when they are added to the national organ donor waiting list informing them of the program. This provides yet another "support" option for transplant patients. *See Appendix (I) for further information.*

CHAPTER TWENTY-TWO

SIDE EFFECTS OF IMMUNOSUPPRESSION

Nothing in life is to be feared. It is only to be understood.
-Marie Curie

At six months post transplantation I began experiencing excessive hair loss on my head. To me this new symptom seemed incongruous in view of the fact that I was still experiencing excessive hair growth everywhere else on my body. I lost approximately fifty-five percent of the hair on my head. This contingency forced me to be creative with the use of my blow dryer and even more so with my hair styling, to give the illusion of hair. Besides, if I were to lose all my hair I would be in vogue. I also consoled myself with the fact that I still had all my teeth.

My hair loss was treated with the use of Rogaine®. I avoided using harsh shampoos and conditioners and used a detangler. I was instructed to pat dry my hair with a towel and use my blow dryer on a limited basis and on the cool setting. I slept with a hairnet to avoid additional hair loss and I also used a detangler comb or brush when styling my hair. I used a minimal amount of sculpting foam and very little hair spray.

I also experienced swollen ankles from sitting at work and a partial tear of my left Achilles tendon. I spent my free time trying to stay cool during some of the hottest pre-summer months ever recorded in Florida. I was also plagued by constant fatigue brought on by a combination of heat, humidity and my medications. In my seventh and eighth months post transplantation I began experiencing swollen and bleeding gums, hypertension, broken blood vessels in my eyes, and gastroesophageal reflux [(GERD) (backing up of stomach acids into the esophagus producing heartburn)].

To avoid infections, my swollen bleeding gums were treated by brushing my teeth three times a day, flossing twice a day, followed by rinsing my mouth with diluted Hydrogen Peroxide®, and a second rinse with an antibacterial mouth wash. To alleviate the reflux and heartburn, I was advised to avoid fatty and fried foods, chocolate, peppermint, bananas, drinking tomato and citrus juices, alcohol, carbonated beverages, coffee, spicy foods and wearing tight fitting clothing. I was also advised to wait for at least one to two hours after eating before lying down. Surprisingly, I was advised to drink a lot of sweet iced tea, which amazingly proved to be of great benedit by alleviated my symptoms within a short time.

The time had come to discontinue the use of the Cytovene® (antiviral). Shortly thereafter I experienced an eruption of Herpes Zoster at one side of my mouth. For this I was treated with Acyclovir® (antiviral) capsules at a very high dose.

Then came the onset of gout, yet another side effect of my medications. The gout affected my thumbs, index fingers and wrists. Sometimes the symptoms were so severe that I could not open jars, make my bed, tie my shoelaces, button my shirt, or even pick up anything which weighed more than the receiver of a telephone. Also, my teeth became temperature sensitive. I could no longer drink cold liquids without the use of a straw. For that reason I adopted the habit of carrying a supply of straws in my handbag. I was also still experiencing excessive hair growth. For this reason I was obliged to continue with my "defurring" with the help of Sally Hansen® hair removal products to avoid looking like an ape.

Yet another side effect of my immunosuppressive therapy is hyperlipidemia which is experienced by 50 percent of all transplant recipients. These clinically high lipid levels (cholesterol and triglycerides) are also affected by the use of beta-blockers, diuretics, diet, obesity, and older age. High lipid levels may cause atherosclerosis and increased cardiovascular morbidity and mortality, and may also contribute to impaired renal function. Keloids, body odor and yellowing of the whites of the eyes and a constant runny nose are other possible side effects of long-term steroid use.

Transplant patients may be at higher risk for developing malignancies. These malignancies include: non-Hodgkin's lymphoma, Kaposi's sarcoma, and cancers of the skin and cervix. The majority of post transplant tumors, however, are low-grade malignancies which are amenable to treatment. Transplant patients are therefore advised to examine themselves for signs of lesions, suspicious growths, discoloration of the skin, swollen lymph nodes, and slow healing wounds.

Women are advised to have regular Mammograms and Papanicolaou (PAP) smears (at six month intervals), and men should have regular prostate examinations and determination of Prostatic Specific Antigen (PSA) levels. Because of immunosuppression female transplant recipients are at a particularly high risk for contracting disorders of the cervix or sexually transmitted diseases. Some of these diseases and viruses are: Acquired Immune Deficiency Syndrome (AIDS), Chlamydia, Genital Herpes, Gonorrhea, Human Immune Deficiency Virus (HIV), Human Papillomavirus (HPV), Pelvic Inflammatory Disease (PID), and Syphilis. *See Glossary for more detailed information.*

Female patients who are sexually active must be extremely careful and practice safe sex. Men can be carriers of viruses and diseases which may be asymptomatic to the male, but could prove harmful to the female genitals and reproductive organs. Additionally, the male genital anatomy is so different from the females that there are some viruses for which the male cannot be tested!

In my ninth month post transplantation I experienced irregular monthly periods and extremely tender and enlarged breasts. My transplant coordinator assured me that these were also common symptoms experienced by female transplant patients.

Other symptoms from my medications included weakness and pain amplification. Pain amplification means that if I hurt myself, the pain would be much more intense than normal and would last for a longer period of time. Thin skin was yet another side effect of my medications. My skin became so thin that you could see networks of green-appearing veins quite clearly as though my skin were transparent. Green is definitely not my color. I felt much like Kermit The Frog® did, when he sang "It's not easy being green...."

Broken blood vessels and painful lumps on the palms of my hands and soles of my feet were also new experiences. As a result of these symptoms, I found it difficult to drive, or perform any task requiring the use of my hands or feet. I also contracted yet another in a long line of urinary tract infections. The infection this time was identified as E.coli and was resistant to all the antibiotics with which I had previously been treated.

Initially, I was told that I would have to be treated with antibiotics via IV, twice a day, every day, for seven to ten days. After my appointment with Dr. Lee, he consulted with a physician in the Department of Infectious Diseases. The physician consulted recommended the use of an oral medication by the name of Macrodantin® (nitrofurantoin mac 100 mg). Needless to say I was greatly relieved because each time I am placed on antibiotics, they react in a certain way, altering my Coumadin® level, and making my blood too thin.

This change necessitates a trip to the Coumadin® Clinic to have my level checked and the dosage adjusted. Maintaining the level within normal range prevents severe bleeding, or clotting my transplanted kidney. Every month I had blood drawn for a PT and International Normalization Ratio (INR) (normal range 2.5-3.5) performed. A patient's INR level is maintained at a low density if they are afflicted with pulmonary embolism, deep vein thrombosis and cardiac disease. A patient's INR level is maintained at a high density if they have had a pacemaker implanted. I was instructed to limit my intake of green leafy vegetables high in Vitamin K (promotes clotting) content, such as: cabbage, cauliflower, tea, and alcohol (promotes thinning of the blood).

Once I had completed my course of Macrodantin®, however, I noticed the return of the foul smell in my urine. I decided not to worry until the results of my latest urinalysis and culture and sensitivity were available. I telephoned Dr. Lee for the results.

At this point in my life I know more about diet and exercise than I ever did. A direct result of this is the fact that I am taking better care of myself than when I was in my twenties. By a kidney patients' standards, I was doing very well and living life one day at a time and each day as though it were my last.

Outwardly, most kidney patients appear to be in good health, but this obvious benefit could also work against you. Along with my friends and co-workers I would sometimes forget how weak I was. This is unfortunate because everyone expects you to give one hundred percent and you in turn push yourself to extremes to meet their expectations. Ultimately, this could be detrimental.

Relationships will continue to be the same. If you act as though everything is all right, it will be. Family members, friends, neighbors and co-workers will take their cue from you. I began a self exploration and I discovered that I had everything I needed for my health, happiness and success within myself. If I lacked anything, I believed that Heavenly Father would provide. Let go and let God!

It was essential for me that goals were set, outlined step by step and accomplished. While I was engaged in accomplishing goals or in the service of others, I had little time to worry about my circumstances or feel sorry for yourself. While a certain amount of self pity may be a normal human trait, I was very careful not to allow myself to wallow in it. In this way, I avoided falling into deep depression. Frankly, I had enough to deal with without the addition of depression.

My kidney transplant had such a direct impact on my body, mind, and outlook that I was changed immeasurably. Little things no longer bothered me. I vowed to extract every ounce of enjoyment I could from life. I began wearing my more expensive pieces of jewelry on a regular basis rather than saving them for special occasions. I thought every day of my new life was such a special occasion. My diet also changed from the standpoint of not liking a great majority of foods I enjoyed in the past. Unfortunately, I have acquired new tastes, among these is a craving for hot fudge sundaes.

Craving sweets was the most confusing change of all because they were never among my favorite things therefore I rarely ate them. These changes in diet were attributed to two factors. The first was that the medications caused most foods to taste bitter. The second, which may sound strange to a non-transplant recipient, was cravings being transmitted to the recipient from the donor organ. After several discussions with other transplant recipients, we discovered that we were all experiencing cravings for foods that we previously detested. Some recipients were also experiencing changes in feelings and even claim to acquire talents they never had before. I, myself, can vouch for the food cravings. The rest, I am not qualified to comment on. I did read an article regarding transplant recipients who received donated organs from a donor who died from a severe allergy to nuts. One recipient could eat nuts without event, while the other developed an allergy to nuts. I do know that this phenomenon is very real and experienced by many recipients. In my opinion, this phenomenon has not been sufficiently researched or documented and certainly warrants it.

Stress is the one thing that all transplant patients are told to avoid. As everyone is aware, this is not easily accomplished. The following is a list of stress relievers that worked for me. Have a support system in place. Talking about your health problem with relatives, friends, support group or mentor is a vital part of the healing process. Attend stress management seminars. Acquire new hobbies. Get involved in your community. Listen to music. Read a book. Call old friends. Learn to paint or play a musical instrument. Plant a tree or flowers and watch them grow. Practice breathing slowly. Go on a picnic. Go see a movie and eat popcorn (unsalted). Feed the birds in the park. Say, "yes," when invited out. Do not stay at home and mope. Get involved!

Remember, you are the best at being you there is. Strive for excellence not perfection. Stop saying negative things to yourself. Look at problems as challenges and look at challenges differently. Pay attention to your appearance. Remember that stress is an attitude. Maintain your weight. Unclutter your life. Change the things about your life that you do not really enjoy. You do not need other people's approval. Do not look for happiness in others, seek it within yourself. The only person who can reject you is you. Do everything in moderation. To dream of what you wish is to waste what you are. Rebuilt your life on your positive traits. We are not perfect, but there are parts of us that are excellent. Visualize yourself winning!

A technique to decrease stress that is gaining popularity is Guided Imagery. Guided imagery is an audio tool specifically designed to help people relieve anxiety, anger, pain, insomnia and medical or surgical procedures. This tool works by telling a story with soothing music in the background. This allows the listener to retreat to a place in their imagination where they feel safe, secure and protected, where they are encouraged to work through their feelings of anger, fear, and negativity. Guided imagery works because it provides the listener the ability to take an active part in their own care. Be aware that guided imagery must not be considered an alternative to medical or surgical treatment. For further information call Diane Tusek, RN, BSN, at the Cleveland Clinic Foundation phone: (440)944-9292, fax: (440)944-1830.

TWENTY-THREE

TOTAL HIP REPLACEMENT

> *Nearly all men die of their medicines, and not of their illnesses.*
> **-Moliere, La Malade Imaginaire**

At ten months post transplantation I was again afflicted with yet another E.coli infection. The medication of choice in this instance was Amikacin® administered via injections. I did, however, continue to experience frequent bladder infections after this incident. I was then referred to a Urologist to rule out the possibility of a mechanical problem which may require surgical repair. If this was not the case, I would then be classified as a patient who is very susceptible to infections on immunosuppression. Fortunately this could be corrected by placing me on chronic antibiotic therapy (a daily, low dose of antibiotics, probably for the rest of my life).

Another new symptom to make its appearance was right hip pain, which was initially thought to be bursitis. Unfortunately, I fell, exacerbating the pain and precipitating a trip to the ER. Standard x-rays performed revealed nothing of my true condition. Given my medical history an MRI followed to be sure nothing was overlooked. The MRI technician tried to convince me that he could "sweet talk" me through the MRI without the use of sedation. On the first two attempts I could feel my anxiety level rising and my body tensing. A nurse offered to hold my hand and talk me through the scan. Although reluctant, I agreed to a third attempt.

This time I closed my eyes before I approached the MRI machine so I could not, at any time, see where I was in relation to the machine. I placed my left hand on my chest and extended my right hand over my head and held the nurse's hand very tightly. I concentrated solely on the nurse's touch as she stroked my right arm. Before I knew it, the scans were over. I experienced a huge sense of pride in myself for having survived an MRI without sedation. Of course, at no time during the scan was my head actually in the machine.

The MRI revealed that I had avascular necrosis (degeneration of bone, cartilage or soft tissues surrounding the joints) of both hips. Avascular necrosis can be caused by a bad injury or long-term use of alcohol or steroids, which can reduce the blood supply to the bone. When the bone dies (necrosis), the joint will decay. It was believed that in my particular case, the avascular necrosis was caused by both the lack of calcium experienced during hemodialysis treatments and by long-term steroid use. The orthopaedic surgeon, Dr. Jennifer Pereira, also discovered what appeared to be fractures at the top of both femoral heads (ball at the top of the femur [long bone of the thigh]). Dr. Pereira's recommendation was no weight bearing on the right hip, the use of crutches for four weeks, followed by re-x-ray. If at re-x-ray, there was no sign of improvement, the pain became worse, or the hip collapsed, my only option then would be total hip replacement. *See Appendix (J) for further information.* Much like the proverbial drowning man I grasped at the offered straw and tried the bed rest. I felt that I had lost enough already and did not want to give up my hip without a fight.

Later that evening I was visiting David Anthony and sharing with him the outcome of my appointment with Dr. Pereira. I asked to use his bathroom, and with his usual rapier whit, he replied, "No! My bathroom is not handicapped accessible." Of course, I felt obliged to point out the fact that he should be nicer to me, because he was meddling with a future bionic woman with the potential to squash him like a bug.

Initially, the pain in my right hip was sharp, stabbing, and only occurred with weight bearing. Within a few days it converted into a constant ache which traveled down my femur (long bone of the thigh), including my knee, then down my tibia (shin). I could no longer cross my right leg over my left, and coughing and rolling over in bed intensified the pain.

Although my hip pain was not improving I still had a difficult time making the decision to proceed with the total right hip replacement. Of course I know now that I was experiencing denial, and I had almost convinced myself that I would improve and not have to part with my hip. My period of denial was short lived, however, because the pain kept intensifying and was a constant reminder that the hip was deteriorating. I was forced to accept the fact that a decision had to be made and some action had to be taken to put an end to the debilitating pain.

I telephoned my transplant surgeon, Dr. Taber to apprise him of the latest developments with my health and have my medical record updated. It was my practice to check with and get Dr. Taber's advice before making any decisions concerning my health. I asked him how common was the occurrence of avascular necrosis among transplant patients. Dr. Taber assured me that avascular necrosis was quite common among transplant patients or patients on extended steroid use.

We discussed my symptoms in great detail, whereupon he advised me to proceed with the hip replacement as soon as possible. He also said that he had seen patients living in terrible pain for extended periods of time before deciding to have the surgery performed. Such was their relief after surgery, they were literally rejuvenated, and regretted bitterly not having the hip replaced sooner. I could not continue to live in such agony or on pain medication forever.

I could not believe this was happening to me. I felt as though I was stuck on a ride at an amusement park and could not get off. I prayed that I would awaken to discover it was just a bad dream. To make matters worse, I awoke one morning to find that I had a film on my left contact lens, and as it was my custom, I removed my lenses and cleaned them both. I replaced the left lens only to find the film was still there. I repeated the cleaning process several times and each time the film remained. Finally, I threw the disposable lenses away and replaced them both with new ones, but still the film still remained.

This could only mean one thing, the problem was not with my left lens but with my eye. Having already endured so many things going wrong with my poor little body, my heart sank and my stomach felt as though it was a clenched fist. I immediately made an appointment to have my eyes examined.

The vision through my left eye gave the illusion that there was a smudge of Vaseline® on my lens, or I was looking through a window pane during a heavy rainfall. I could no longer read through my left eye, and though cloudy, I could still discern objects and colors. At the end of my eye examination the ophthalmologist confirmed my worst suspicions. Yes, I indeed had a cataract in my left eye which would only become worse and would require surgical removal. Yes, there was also the beginning of a cataract in my right eye as well.

He continued by explaining that the human eyes are composed of mainly water and protein. The protein is arranged in such a way to allow the passage of light through, and to focus on the retina. These proteins sometimes clump together, clouding the lens. This is called a cataract. It was my hope that I would not have to deal with this contingency for a few more months. Besides, the cataracts were not the "hot issue" in my life at the time. *See Appendix (K) for further information.*

The new complication with the cataract threw me off blance and once again forced me to regroup. If regrouping were an Olympic event I would win the gold. I had only just come to terms with the avascular necrosis, then found myself having to cope with my lost vision and future cataract surgery. If the day ever came when I found myself dealing with only one crisis I am not sure I would know how to act. My friend Sarah once said that she endured a period of thirty days without incident and waited with fevered anticipation for the bolt of lightening. On the thirty-first day she experienced a mishap and immediately relaxed. I now understand her predicament exactly.

I was plagued by the thought that I was losing my vision permanently. These thoughts produced fear and anxiety and I could only sleep with all the lights on in my apartment including the television. It took me approximately two weeks to come to terms with this new development. I have to confess that I began to question whether the kidney transplant was in fact worth all that I was currently experiencing. The answer, is still a resounding yes.

Due to PKD, the one constant in my life became change. I found myself regrouping each time a new side effect or complication of my disease occurred. I became extremely skilled at rolling with the punches; a fact of life for most transplant patients. I was forced to come to terms with the fact that my hip was not improving. I was unable to walk or drive because the pain had become unbearable.

I rescheduled my appointment with Dr. Pereira for an earlier date. Another MRI was performed for comparison with my previous scan. The comparison revealed a significant amount of degeneration since the last MRI was performed. I could no longer avoid the inevitable. I requested the first available surgery date, which was scheduled before I left Dr. Pereira's office.

I felt as though a weight had been lifted. Having a plan made all the difference in the world. As I was leaving Dr. Pereira's office I asked her what the possibility was of having a "turbo model" hip implanted. I could not resist asking whether or not I could walk through an airport metal detector without causing it to alarm. She looked at me, shook her head and laughed.

With the surgery scheduled, I began making preparations and leaving everything at my apartment in readiness. With help, I managed to accomplish my Christmas shopping, the mailing of my Christmas cards, and the decorating.

As a matter of routine, immunosuppressed patients are premedicated prior to surgery to reduce the risk of infection. I was admitted to the hospital three days prior to my surgery so I could be pre-medicated with antibiotics. If an infection should occur in my new hip, it would have to be removed. I would be confined to a hospital bed on antibiotic therapy via IV for a six-week period. At the end of this time, another hip replacement would be attempted. If this failed I would remain with a "flail hip" and a limp for the rest of my life. A "flail hip" is what remains after the prosthesis is removed. In other words, a joint that does not articulate, or a joint that does not have a femoral head (ball).

This type of hip is held in place by the muscles and there is a certain amount of free movement. A patient with a flail hip joint will never graduate to using a cane, and will have to use either crutches or a walker for the rest of their lives.

I have a limited amount of accesses in the way of veins, and those precious few are very delicate. A Peripherally Inserted Central Catheter ([PICC-line], type of permanent access with two ports used for blood drawing and IV's) had to be placed in my right upper inner arm. Placement of a PICC line is ultrasound-guided and because the vein is deep-seated a contrast or dye is injected to enhance the visibility of the vein. After placement of the PICC line and a three-day course of antibiotics I was ready for surgery. Back in my room after the hip replacement, I felt quite well and in little discomfort. This was due to the epidural and the PCA pump (patient controlled analgesic/pain killer) which administered a pre-measured quantity of Dilaudid®. The medication was pre-measured to eliminate the danger of overdosing. This method of pain control provided a steady level of pain relief via IV with just the push of a button.

The PCA pump and I bonded. A few days later the epidural was removed and the pump was disconnected. I was then switched to a twelve-hour-acting oral analgesic, a narcotic named Oxycontin®. For me, the pain became excruciating. My pain control regimen consisted of two Oxycontin® tablets a day and one to two Percocet® every four to six hours as needed to control break-through pain. For the remainder of my hospital stay I consumed a considerable amount of Percocet® for pain control. TED® elastic hose had to be worn all day to reduce the risk of blood clots in my legs.

A huge foam wedge was placed between my legs to keep them apart. A bar (trapeze) was hanging over my bed so I could lift myself to change positions. When I asked if the foam wedge indicated that I had become a Greenbay Packers® fan, a "cheese head," my question was met with blank stares. I guess I was surrounded by non-sports fans.

The day following surgery physical therapists helped me out of bed and into the "hip chair" for a period of one hour. The second day after surgery, the physical therapists began my exercise regimen, to increase circulation and build the strength of the muscles in my calf, thigh, buttocks and hip. I could not believe the severity of the pain. I cried uncontrollably. I asked if their other patients were in as much pain, and I told the therapists that I would rather have another kidney transplant than have another hip replacement.

Every day I was quizzed on my restrictions, which were: do not bend my hip more than 90 degrees (bend over), do not cross my operated leg over my other leg (do not cross the midline), and do not turn my operated leg inward (pigeon-toed). I was taught how to get out of bed, stand, sit, and walk with the aid of a walker so I could perform these actions safely. I was assured that I could return to most normal activities but to avoid squatting, hyper-extension (extreme extension) and anything which would cause a high-impact on my hip. Extreme extension could cause subluxation (partial dislocation). I asked if bungee jumping was out of the question.

While still in the hospital my friend Mike and his son came to visit me, both wearing rubber gloves. They advised me that there was a Contact Isolation warning posted on my door and they were instructed by the nurse to wear gloves. My first emotion was embarrassment, then I was filled with a certain amount of concern because I had not been on isolation that morning. Since I had blood and urine samples taken that morning for testing, and I was placed on isolation that afternoon, I wondered if my test results had revealed yet another infection.

When Mike and his son were leaving, they were given instructions on how to remove their gloves, where to dispose of them, and also instructed on the use of the antibacterial/antiviral solution which was contained in a dispenser on the wall just outside my door.

As soon as my visitors left I asked the nurse why I had been placed on isolation. I was informed that the Infections Diseases Nurse reviewed my chart and discovered that six months previously I did have a Multiple Drug Resistant (MDR) Bacteria. After treatment, three negative results are required to be removed from contact isolation. To the best of their knowledge, I did not have an active infection. Being placed on isolation was merely a precautionary measure and hospital policy. *See Appendix (L) for further information on isolation and MDR Bacteria*. Prior to my release from the hospital the Case Manager saw to my discharge needs which were: home health care, physical therapy, and equipment (walker, grabber, extended toilet seat).

I could not accomplish anything unaided and apart from my physical therapy and walking to the bathroom I spent most of my time lying down and taking a considerable amount of pain medication. My back ached horribly. I relied heavily on the equipment I was provided and I must confess that I did not always adhere to my exercise regimen. Although my recovery was progressing at a normal rate, it was not fast enough for me. I was anxious to return to work. I was filled with a huge sense of frustration. This was the second consecutive Christmas that I found myself totally dependent on the help of friends and David Anthony.

Not being able to drive or take a short walk drove me crazy. I felt claustrophobic, as though the walls of my apartment were closing in on me. I read as much as possible to avoid watching too many hours of television. I still managed to develop an addiction to the Biography and Discovery channels, and The Essence of Emeril® became my favorite cooking show.

Christmas day arrived and David Anthony and I along with his dog Penny and my bird Jake had a quiet but wonderful day. We enjoyed breakfast followed by the opening of our presents, watched a movie and napped. We then enjoyed a short drive followed by an early dinner. David Anthony having to work the following morning left early for bed. I made several phone calls to family and friends, and stayed up late reading a book I had received as a Christmas present.

All too soon New Year's Eve was upon us and David Anthony and I spend a little quality time with friends. We ushered in the new year at my apartment, by watching "the ball" go down in Central Park on television. This also was a quiet day but very enjoyable. The following morning I telephoned Sarah to wish her a Happy New Year. During our conversation we began reflecting on the events of the past year. Sarah said, "Given the events of your life during the past three years, you are not going to have anything to look forward to when you grow old." "You already have your Medicare Card, Disabled Persons Parking Permit, right hip replaced, and soon cataract surgery on both eyes." I quickly responded, "I could always wear purple, invest in a rocking chair or perhaps a shawl." We discussed our new year's resolutions, and hoped that the new year would be better for both of us.

After several weeks of therapy it was time to graduate from a walker to a cane. I selected an adjustable aluminum cane. When I arrived home and proceeded to use my cane, I came to the realization that all canes are not created equal. The cane I had selected was too tall for me and was already adjusted to its lowest level. Fortunately, I was not presented with any resistance when I returned the cane in exchange for one more appropriate for my height. The guidelines for selecting a cane are: stand upright on a firm, flat surface. Wear the style shoes you plan to wear when using your cane. Allow your arm to hang down. The cane is the proper length when the handle of the cane touches the inside of your wrist where it meets your palm.

The switch from the walker to the cane afforded me a greater degree of mobility because the walker was cumbersome to use in an apartment which was not handicap accessible. By this I mean that I had to enter and exit rooms sideways because with the exception of my front door, the walker was wider than the remaining doors in my apartment. To avoid cabin fever, with the use of my cane, I would stand outside my apartment door for a few minutes to gaze at the sky and feel the warmth of the sun.

Prior to my sixth week of physical therapy, David Anthony collected my mail. After six weeks of physical therapy, I had achieved a certain degree of proficiency with my cane and was strong enough to walk to the mailbox and collect the mail myself. I was so proud of myself. This in my estimation was quite an accomplishment. I had come a long way. From the time my illness became apparent, I promised myself to celebrate every one of my little successes. I have, and will continue to do so.

For me, the new year started with a bang. It began with my birthday celebration complete with presents and dinner at my favorite restaurant with David Anthony. Being taken out to dinner was particularly enjoyable because of my confinement in my apartment for such an extended period of time. The birthday present I gave myself was a new look which took the form of a short haircut. I had lost so much hair that I looked ungroomed. I consider every birthday post transplantation a hallmark event and I intend to celebrate each one to the hilt.

The following week, Dr. Taber decreased my immunosuppressant medication by fifty percent and I was told that during the month of February we would begin tapering the other steroids. This would certainly help with my weight loss. This was especially good news. I had managed to gain weight because of lying down for such a great deal of time and eating out of boredom. I was happy indeed that the new year had so far brought me nothing but good news.

I spoke too soon, however. Added to the fact that my night vision has been deteriorating over the last three years and with the addition of the cataract in my left eye, I had a halo effect around all street and automobile lights at night. I discontinued driving at night and in the early morning because my perception and judgement were slightly impaired.

My hip, however, was doing so well that on my last visit with Dr. Pereira she released me from home health care and physical therapy. She also told me I could begin driving again, and resume work. The icing on top of my cake was the fact that I had begun to lose weight. There was a new song being sung in my apartment, "I'm Still Standing, Yeah, Yeah, Yeah..." As to my relationship with David Anthony, I could only hope that it will grow and endure.

TWENTY-FOUR

AND THE BEAT GOES ON....

*I'd gone through life believing in the strength and competence
of others; never in my own. Now, dazzled,
I discovered that my capacities were real.
It was like finding a fortune in the lining of an old coat.*

-Joan Mills

Due to the cataract, the vision in my left eye was deteriorating at what I felt was a very rapid rate. I called for an ophthalmology appointment to discuss my surgical options, hoping that I could have the cataract surgically repaired in the not too distant future. At the same time, my right hip was healing at such a rapid rate that I hardly felt the need to use my cane. I had just begun to feel confident and was preparing to return to work, when I began experiencing uncomfortable twinges in my left hip.

I was amazed at the degree of deterioration which occurred within 7 days. History was indeed repeating itself. The pain in my left hip became so intense that once again I was forced to take analgesics and I could not walk without the aid of a walker. Yes, the very same walker that I had stored in my closet and hoped never to use again.

When I telephoned Dr. Pereira's office I was told that it had already been established that I have avascular necrosis in both hips and that surgery could not be scheduled until I had achieved three months post operative status.

I had to wait a month in pain before the other hip surgery could be performed. After my second hip replacement I would have a matched set of scars curving from my hip and running down both thighs. I was racking up the scars as though they were frequent flyer miles. Good grief! I really was turning into the "Bionic Woman."

Upon sharing my news with David Anthony, he said that I should count my blessings that I was not an automobile, otherwise I would be totaled. When I asked him if he was planning on trading me in, he replied that he had already attempted to do but could not find a dealership that would accept me. He was stuck with me, he said. I through we were lucky to be stuck with each other. I was also stuck with the knowledge that I could do nothing but wait until my second hip replacement could be scheduled.

Dr. Pereira was surprised to hear that I had requested a refill on my pain medication because I was doing so well on my last visit. She was advised by her PA (physician's assistant) that my left hip was degenerating and I was unable to return to work as anticipated. An appointment was immediately scheduled for an x-ray of the left hip. The x-ray confirmed the degeneration. The left total hip replacement was immediately scheduled.

The speed at which the left hip had degenerated was staggering. The degree of pain was worse than before. This time I felt no reluctance whatsoever toward parting with my hip. In fact, the surgery date seemed eons away. My thoughts were consumed with how wonderful it would be to live pain free. Lucky for me, the right hip healed very rapidly because I needed to rely on it for support. I was forced to shift my weight to the right hip in order to favor the left.

The pain became so severe that I felt capable of ripping my left hip out myself in order to relieve the pain. My attention was divided by counting the days until my hip replacement surgery and concern for the cataract in my left eye. Five days after my initial consultation with the ophthalmologist, however, I had the cataract removed and a permanent lens implanted. I also had Lasix surgery performed at the same time to correct my vision for distance.

Directly after the surgery I could see clearly without the aid of glasses or contact lenses. In a matter of days my left eye had healed and I enjoyed perfect vision. I could hardly wait for the cataract in my right eye to mature so I could have the surgery performed in that eye as well. As the old saying goes, "Be careful what you wish for..."

Several weeks later I had my left total hip replacement. This time I knew what to expect and was only to anxious to see the physical therapist and begin the healing process. I still had all the equipment from my last surgery and my discharge needs were for home health care and physical therapy only.

One of the main differences between the two hip replacements was the closure of the incisions. A "plastic closure" utilizing sutures was used for the closure of the incision from the first hip replacement. This is the type generally used by plastic surgeons and produces a much thinner and neater-looking scar. Patients can request a "plastic closure." Staples were used for the closure of my second hip replacement. Apart from the fact that the staples frequently caught on my clothing and bedding, this type of closure left me with a wider and more pronounced scar.

I now had a matching set of cobalt hips. One of my friends asked me with tongue-in-cheek if he could consult with me before he went fishing. I responded by saying that I could certainly be of help relative to weather changes but I could not predict the tides. Everyone is a comedian.

While recovering from my left hip surgery I began experiencing several other problems. One was acne, for which my transplant coordinator suggested the use of Calamine® lotion which I applied and left on my face overnight. This regimen was very effective. The medication-induced gout which previously attacked the joints in my hands now affected all the joints in my body. My muscles and tendons were also becoming affected.

Once again I was tested for Lupus and arthritis with negative results. A trip to the Department of Physical Medicine and Rehabilitation resulted in a diagnosis of fibromyalgia which is a painful muscular-type of rheumatism that can also affect the joints and has the potential of producing a host of other problems.

My joint symptoms were relieved only to a minimal degree by limiting the quantity of red meat I ate. Eating too large a quantity of red meat raises the uric acid level which can cause gout or arthritic-type symptoms. I was also instructed to discontinue the use of Lipitor® which interacted with my other medications and caused a certain amount of my joint symptoms. My symptoms could not be relieved altogether because the majority of my discomfort was caused by my fibromyalgia. It was then that I discovered Flexaril® (muscle relaxant), as well as Glucosamine® and Chondriton® , and combining them with exercise, my pain was alleviated. As part of my recovery I was required to walk a certain amount each day. I referred to my gradually-increased daily walks as taking my hips on a test drive. Soon I was walking without visible signs of a limp.

A few weeks before I was scheduled to return to work a cloud descended upon my right eye much as it did previously with my left. In my life, history has made a habit of repeating itself. The scenario was the same, and of course a few days later I had the cataract from my right eye removed and a permanent lens implanted. Soon full vision was restored to both eyes and each day seemed like a new gift. Lights were brighter and colors were considerably more vibrant than I remembered. I wore sunglasses frequently until my eyes could adjust to light.

My vision seemed a great deal crisper and clearer. I noticed the most minute of imperfections in objects around me. Much like a child seeing everything for the first time, I was overwhelmed by everything I saw. It seemed as though I was being besieged by too much information for my eyes to process. This took some getting used to. It was not long before I adjusted to my new vision and enjoyed the freedom from glasses and contacts. I was also able to drive at night.

While at home recovering from eye surgery my friend Ken visited me. He asked how I could possibly have lenses implanted in my eyes. My response was, "After two kidney transplants, and two hip replacements, what's a lens?" Kenneth laughed and replied, "I see your point."

TWENTY-FIVE

ADVICE, ADVANCES,
SHORTAGE OF ORGAN DONORS

You may have to fight a battle more than once to win it.
-**Margaret Thatcher**

Through dealing with my own challenges I learned that despite a patient's intelligence level and knowledge of the medical field, when dealing with his/her own health issues, the stress created can cloud your judgement. For this reason I cannot emphasize enough the importance of transplant patients educating themselves and taking an active part in their own health care. The members of your health care team are human, therefore subject to mistakes along with the rest of humanity. These mistakes could prove costly.

One way in which the transplant patient can minimize the risk of mistakes is to ask questions. For example, before taking any medications ask what they are. Ask why they are being prescribed and what specific benefit is expected. Avail yourself of every possible resource including public and medical libraries to obtain information relative to your specific health condition. Request explanations for what you do not understand. I also learned that there is a normal process that takes place in every transplant patient's life. We all experience the steps of denial, anger, depression, low morale or self-esteem, desire to die, acceptance, and finally change of attitude.

For me, the acceptance and change of attitude phases occurred when I was told I had an excellent chance of surviving my kidney disease. I became possessed by a will to live and resolved to do whatever was required to survive. The sad truth is that all transplant patients lose a lot, and once lost, cannot be recovered. We have to preserve what we have left at all cost, and do the best we can with what we have left. If I have any advice to give it is this, explore all your options thoroughly with your physician, and together with your physician make the decision as to what type of treatment is best for you.

Take into account your lifestyle and financial situation before making any decisions. Do not allow experimentation unless you are out of options. Select someone you can trust, a spouse, family member or close friend and appoint them as a healthcare suggorate to help you make intelligent decisions relative to your health care. I say this because the psychological toll of a life threatening disease is of the extreme. Such is the state of flux in which transplant patients find themselves that many question their values, outlook, and whether or not they have the strength to endure. Avoid making life-altering decisions without help.

Family members and/or spouse may also express emotional difficulty through: extreme anger, inappropriate sense of denial out of ordinary depression, expression of suicide and excessive substance abuse.

Death is a very real possibility both for yourself as well as other transplant recipients with whom you may have forged a friendship. It was suggested to me that I deal with this possibility before I find myself in a situation where I lose a recipient/friend and begin questioning my own mortality.

Other pieces of advice I would like to share is the importance of wearing a MedicAlert® bracelet. To order call 1-800-432-5378. In the event of an emergency, knowing what special medications you are taking would have a direct impact in determining your health care requirements. Ask your physician to consult the Pharmaceutical Research and Manufacturers of America (PhARMA®) directory, and to call the "physicians only number" to inquire if you qualify for any of their Prescription Drug Patient Assistance Programs. *See page 148.*

Before each visit to your physician ask for all the literature available to provide you with what you need to know and what you need to avoid. Never forget to take your list of questions with you to your doctors appointments.

Be very careful of the advice given by well-meaning friends. For example, one friend told me that I was not normal and would never be normal again. That I would not be able to work, take care of myself, buy a home, have a relationship with a member of the opposite sex and certainly would never remarry.

I refused to accept this line of thinking, and I have already proven my friend wrong on several counts. Furthermore, anyone who looks at me and sees nothing but my illness is narrow minded in the extreme. In essence what I am being told is that everything I was prior to PKD ceased to exist and all I have become is my disease. I will not allow anyone to place limits on what I can or cannot do. I myself do not know what I am capable of until I try. Setting and accomplishing goals is not age-specific. There is no expiration date.

It is important for patients who lose their allograft to know that hemodialysis and peritoneal dialysis could be viable options for them. They can live long healthy lives on dialysis. Currently, this is especially true because of the latest developments and improvements made in PD. There are new technologies raising peritoneal clearances. New solutions such as Icodextrin® (a glucose polymer acting as a colloid osmotic agent) which may soon replace dextrose in the dialysate.

Dextrose has the advantage of being inexpensive but it causes hyperglycemia, hyperlipidemia, and obesity. Luckily, I did not experience peritoneal membrane damage because Dr. Lee limited my use of the higher concentrations of dextrose. It is my hope that in the not too distant future, advances in medicine would be such that transplantation would no longer be necessary.

Other advances in medicine include, stripping the epithelial layer off of kidneys harvested from pigs and genetically engineering a new epithelial layer using cells from the recipient. In this way the recipient's body can be duped into believing that the transplanted kidney belongs to the recipient. The odds of rejecting the transplanted kidney are minimal, therefore, the recipient takes little or no antirejection medications.

Another area of research is genetically engineering a kidney from healthy cells taken from the unaffected portion of the patient's own kidneys. When the cells begin generating, they are placed in a kidney-shaped mold. Then polymers are used to tell the tissue which way to curve or where to indent, giving the organ its shape. It is predicted that in approximately three years this genetic engineering could be a reality giving new hope to thousands of transplant recipients. Because the kidney is engineered from the recipient's own cells, the body will accept the kidney as its own, eliminating the need for immunosuppressant medications.

The latest and greatest hope in fighting transplant rejection is an FDA-approved medication named daclizumab®, brand name (Zenapax®). This wonder drug is a monoclonal antibody which is bioengineered. Daclizumab® blocks the immune cells from attacking the allograft the first few weeks after transplantation. Daclizumab® is used in conjunction with standard anti-rejection drugs which makes daclizumab® more effective with less side effects. Daclizumab® is administered intravenously within 24 hours before transplantation. Subsequent doses are administered at 2, 4, 6, and 8 weeks post transplantation.

Daclizumab® targets activated T-cells (immune system cells programmed to attack foreign bodies or cells). It prevents the T-cells from harming the transplanted kidney. This medication is unique because of its ability to single out and suppress the T-cells alone, leaving the integrity of the remaining cells of the immune system intact. Daclizumab® has not yet been tested as an antirejection medication for organs other than kidneys!

On the surgical front, a rib is no longer sacrificed to remove a donor organ. Laparoscopic surgery is the latest surgical technique used for organ retrieval.

This is accomplished through several small one-inch incisions in the upper abdominal area. The operation is performed with the use of a camera which is inserted through one of the incisions, while pencil-thin instruments are inserted through the remaining incisions. The kidney is removed through a five-to-seven inch incision extending just below the navel. The benefits of laparoscopic surgery are: less post-operative pain, shorter hospital stay and quicker recovery time.

Transplantation relies heavily on organ donations. There are 35,475 prospective recipients registered for kidney transplants. The names on the waiting lists for transplants is growing because of a shortage of donated organs. For this reason, consideration is being given to offering financial incentives as a means to increase organ donation. This idea is considered by some health care professionals as politically incorrect and not deserving of consideration.

Health care professionals are concerned that they will be perceived as profiting from the tragedy of others. They also fear that the question would be raised as to whether or not every option was explored to save the donor's life. There is also the belief that systems become corrupt with the introduction of money. I myself, am living proof that organ transplants save lives. Needless to say I am an ardent advocate for organ and tissue donation. There is a large segment of the American population who embrace the idea of helping families with funeral expenses or paying a death benefit to maximize life-saving organ donations.

A pilot program to offer donor families a $1000 death benefit to help with funeral expenses has been proposed. There are ethical issues, however, that must first be resolved before this program could become a reality. Nine to ten people on transplant lists die every day. The three main reasons for lack of organ donation are: no signed organ donor cards, patient's family is not asked to donate, and cause of patient's death may have caused the kidneys to become diseased.

There are new federal rules designed to increase organ donation. For example, all hospitals in the U.S. will be required to notify an organ procurement organization (OPO) of all deaths occurring at their facilities. This will allow the OPO the opportunity to determine the suitability of potential organ donors, increasing the contact with families to request organ donation.

There was also a national organ and tissue donation initiative announced by the Clinton administration, implemented by the Department of Health and Human Services, with the goal of increasing by 20 percent, the number of Americans donating organs and tissues. A few of the organizations joining the quest include: The American Medical Association and the American Academy of Family Physicians. These organizations will make donation literature available in their offices. The American Bar Association will discuss organ donation with clients during will preparation. The American Association Health Plans will provide materials to their members. The U.S. Chamber of Commerce will implement outreach programs to their employees and other businesses through the nation. The American Red Cross will expand public awareness to promote organ and tissue donation. Another reason cited for the death of prospective recipients while on the waiting list is reluctance to donate. This reluctance stems from certain moral or philosophical values, and religious beliefs.

Among certain ethnic groups the reasons given for their reluctance to donate organs were: lack of information, religious myths, distrust of health care professionals, fear of premature death and racism. There is also the stigma created by the modern myths. Myths of people being drugged for the purpose of stealing their kidneys. Children in Third World countries kidnaped for their organs which are purchased by wealthy Americans. The wealthy receiving better health care than the poor, and prisoners offering to donate their organs for money. Although research has proven these myths untrue, they have had a negative impact on prospective organ donors by creating anxiety at a subconscious level. Furthermore, organ transplantation is a highly complicated and technical process requiring the use of the highest level surgical facility and surgically trained professionals. Clandestine organ transplantations are an impossibility.

The latest advancement relative to PKD is that scientists have localized the gene responsible for ARPKD to a small region of chromosome 6. Another finding which may lead to clinical trials is a new drug which blocked the activity of a common growth factor receptor (EGFR). This produced a significant reduction in cyst growth and prolonged the life span in an animal model of ARPKD.

Significant changes in the PKD1 gene which cause PKD in different families has been identified. Within any family, the individuals with PKD will have the same change in the PKD1 gene, however, among families with PKD, the changes may be different. The soy protein diet was also discovered to clearly decrease renal cyst volume and improved kidney function in an animal model. Taxol®, was thought to inhibit cyst enlargement, but recent studies have failed to confirm this. Currently, laparoscopic surgery to either partially remove or broadly open the cysts in the kidneys to reduce pain and overall volume is another available option. This surgery requires a hospital stay of three days and produces minimal scarring.

Minority Organ/Tissue Transplant Education Program (MOTTEP), believes that when it comes to saving lives, everyone should be involved. For this reason MOTTEP is trying to change people's attitudes and behavior toward organ donation by implementing community-based, grass roots programs designed to increase the number of minorities who sign donor cards. I do not know what the key might be to solving these religious, moral and philosophical issues, I only know that needless deaths could be prevented through organ donation/recovery.

In 1989, 1,878 people died while on the active national list to receive a cadaveric organ; 749 of these were waiting for kidneys. With the exception of 1998 when cadaveric donation increased 5.6 percent, the number of organ donors in the United States over the last decade approximated 4000-5000 annually. However, the use of living donors has almost doubled in the same time period.

Cadaveric organ recovery currently is still not meeting the demand. This is especially true in minority populations, for this reason, payment to donor families would probably favor minority populations. Studies have shown that the survival rate of an allograft from a living donor is longer than that of a cadaver donor. Benefits to the recipients are avoidance of dialysis or complications associated with ESRD. The donors benefit by experiencing an increased sense of self-worth from donating.

Organ Transplant Donor and Recipient Listing (for all organs) in the U.S.: Number of Organ Donors, Number of Patients Awaiting Transplantation and Number of Patients Who Died Waiting for Transplants.

Time Period			*No. of Patients*	
Year	Total Cadaver Donors for all Organs	Total Patients Awaiting Transplantation for All Organs	Total Patients Died Waiting for All Organs	Total Patients Died Waiting for Kidneys only
1988	4,084	16,026	1,496	736
1989	4,019	19,095	1,669	749
1990	4,512	21,914	1,958	916
1991	4,528	24,719	2,351	974
1992	4,521	29,415	2,573	1,047
1993	4,861	33,394	2,883	1,277
1994	5,100	37,684	3,053	1,365
1995	5,357	43,937	3,414	1,503
1996	5,412	50,130	3,897	1,802
1997	5,478	61,000	4,316	1,991
*1998	*5,081	*41,000	*3,282	*1,594

*Data from Jan.-Aug. 1998.
Source: UNOS Scientific Registry as of 2/3/99.

Living-unrelated third party kidney donations through a Third Party Donor

Registry is increasing each year. This increase is being brought about through the efforts of its many avid supporters, among whom is Thomas G. Peters, M.D., director of the Jacksonville Transplant Center at Methodist Medical Center, who is also a clinical professor of surgery at the University of Florida Health Sciences Center. According to Dr. Peters, third party donation is safe, effective and becoming more acceptable to potential donors due to better pain control techniques and shorter hospital stays. The third party donor is studied and accepted for donation to his/her relative, but is unable to donate a kidney because of ABO or crossmatch incompatibility. This donor in turn is willing to donate his/her kidney to an unrelated recipient in exchange for a healthy kidney for his/her relative. This third party donation is also referred to as "paired exchange" or "donor swapping."

These surgeries would have to occur simultaneously so both recipients could receive a kidney at the same time. The transplant facility would need the capacity to run four operating rooms at the same time (one for each donor and recipient). For this reason, some transplant centers are moving ahead with this type of exchange program while others remain hesitant.

Certain ethical issues have been raised, which include: how would a recipient feel about letting a loved one donate to a complete stranger? Would the emotional benefits gained be as great if donating to a stranger? What if one kidney works, and the other does not? What if potential donors were relieved because they were incompatible, and not feel pressured to donate? What if one donor changes his/her mind after the other recipient has already received the exchanged kidney?

Other provocative questions are: should transplant recipients be eligible to be re-transplanted? Should they then be given higher or lower priority than those who have not been transplanted? The experience by many centers with unrelated kidney donors has been excellent for the transplanted kidney, donor and recipient survival, demonstrating that the benefits far outweigh the risks.

Renal allograft survival is related to recipient race. Antigen expression differs among different populations. Transplants are least available for patients who are transfused, multiparous, and who are immunologically sensitized black women. It is hoped that payment of a death benefit will increase organ donation in populations that donate fewest organs, and need them the most.

While waiting for a chance at a new life, do not fall into the trap of believing that time is running out. This line of thinking causes anger and frustration. Ultimately, too much time is wasted thinking about what you could have accomplished instead of enjoying what you have now.

In the beginning I felt as though I had nothing to offer and was afraid to allow anyone close to me. I feared that they could not deal with my illness, as has happened in the past. I am back working full-time and actively planning to return to college to continue with my education. Never again do I want to be perceived as a liability and not an asset. In retrospect, I would not trade any of my experiences. I see them as opportunities I was presented with to learn and grow. I believe I have emerged a much better, stronger and more confident person.

The many experiences I have shared with my readers are not intended to scare but to educate. If in the beginning I had a better idea of the post transplant variables, the element of surprise and my anger would both have been less intense. It is my hope that in some small way I have made a contribution, and my contribution will be of help to many transplant patients.

Since I no longer require dialysis I have regained three hours every day. I am also free of tubes and machines. I now sing a new tune as I walk around my apartment, just as Pinocchio did when he became a real boy, "There are no strings on me..."

I try to enjoy and not waste a precious moment of my newfound freedom; the freedom for which I paid an exorbitant price. Even today freedom is still a very precious and costly commodity. Every cloud does in fact have a silver lining, though some instances require digging way down deep to find it. Had I not received my kidney I would not be unhappy today. Peritoneal dialysis worked exceptionally well for me and my only medications were: calcium, a multivitamin, and one Epogen® injection a week. My medications did not produce any side effects and I maintained my weight. I also had an excellent energy level and I looked and felt terrific.

Among the many lessons I learned battling PKD is to keep my health challenges in perspective. Not to lose my compassion for others or understanding for the human condition. It is easy to perceive other's problems as petty or trivial while you are fighting for your life. Everything is relative.

Each time I am asked how I managed, especially living alone, my answer is the same. Exercise a lot of faith, prayer, positive mental attitude (50-70 percent of your battle), and a good support system.

I also embarked on a crusade to find out the things in life that made me happy, so I could do those things for myself. Living alone, there are times when there is no one available when I need a hug and to hear the words "Everything is going to be all right." I therefore devised ways to give myself these hugs. One of the ways in which I chose to do this is by taking extra care with my appearance. If I did not take this extra effort on my own behalf, I would see a depressed person who felt badly every time I looked in a mirror. I could not allow myself to become depressed. Making this extra effort made me feel much better mentally, physically and emotionally.

Laughter, is the second item on my list of self-hugs. Learn to laugh at yourself. For example, I laugh because I believe that by the time they are through replacing all my parts I would be much too valuable to throw away. I would absolutely have to be recycled. Its nice to know that I have some value. At least I am worth my weight in chromium cobalt.

Another self-hug is my joining Weight Watchers®. In my opinion it is the easiest and healthiest way to lose and maintain weight. I am back to work full-time, losing weight, feeling good about myself and my new job. I am also fortunate to have dual medical insurance coverage. Medicare is currently my primary insurer because of my kidney transplants. My secondary group insurance coverage through my employer continued throughout my period of disability. When my Medicare coverage stops, my secondary insurer reverts back to being primary and my coverage continues.

Loretta LaRoche from the Mind/Body Institute in Boston says in her talks and video tapes of the same titles: "The Joy of Stress®" and "Humor Your Stress Away®," that we should applaud our lives, and accept ourselves as we are today. We each have to find those individual ways to accomplish this for ourselves.

I am not afraid of dying, but dying without accomplishing the goals I have set for myself and leaving this earth with regrets. It is my prayer that I will be allotted the time necessary to accomplish these goals. If we can adjust our perspective, and use humor, we can overcome even the most challenging aspects of our disease. I believe where there is laughter, there is hope. Remember, laughter is less expensive than therapy.

As to your future. Your future is what you make of it, so make it a good one. *I intend to.*

AFTERWORD

I read this manuscript from several points of view. First and foremost, as a patient who, from age 7 has had her life shaped and controlled by kidney disease and its side effects. Second, as a nursing professional who took nurses training, in part, to facilitate learning how to live with this disease and its effect on my life and third, as someone who loves and deeply respects the author of this wonderful enlightening piece of literature. I found this volume to be a clearly written work that even a young kidney patient would be able to read and understand. The sense of humor, courage and spirituality of Donna Pollard shines from every page.

The insightful and thorough research that she put into this work, along with her self knowledge, which she has come to on her journey through the years of this disease, make this a "teaching manual" which, in my opinion, should be required reading by every patient, health care professional, family member and even close friends of those touched by any form of kidney disease. To the teams of doctors, nurses, Lab Technicians and other medical professionals who brought my friend through this long, trying journey (you know who you are), I dedicate the following:

As she walked the path of illness,
the Lord stretched out his arms,
and whispered softly to her spirit,
I'll protect you from all harm.

Men and women I have sent,
with gentle hands and caring faces,
who have searched for all the answers,
knowledge gained in diverse places.

Tirelessly they are daily working,
as a team to cure her ills,
with the miracle of dialysis,
and transplantation and of pills.

Now she walks with head uplifted,
renewed legs support her frame,
and a kidney now perfected,
given by one of unknown name.

Now the teams of medical professionals,
to other patients turn their care,
and she'll ask her Heavenly Father,
"bless them daily" is her prayer.

-Ellen W. Bryan

118

GLOSSARY OF MEDICAL TERMS

Adult Onset.
The onset or beginning of a disease or condition after an individual achieves adulthood.

Analgesic.
An agent that alleviates pain without causing loss of consciousness.

Aneurysm.
A sac formed by the dilation of the wall of an artery, vein, or the heart; it is filled with fluid or clotted blood.

Angiogram.
An x-ray of blood vessels.

Antibody.
Protein substances developed by the body, in response to the presence of an antigen which has been administered parenterally or has otherwise gained access to the body.

Anticardiolipin/ Antiphospholipid antibody.
Antibody associated with thrombosis or clotting disorder.

Anticoagulant.
Commonly referred to as a blood thinner.

Antigen.
A substance which induces the formation of antibodies. An antigen may be introduced into the body or it may be formed within the body.

Antecubital fossa.
Bend in the arm opposite or in front of the elbow.

Antifungal.
Destroying or preventing the growth of fungi.

Antiglobulin.
A precipitin which precipitates globulin.

Antihypertensive.
Medication used to lower the blood pressure.

Arterioles.
Minute arteries, especially those which, at its distal end, leads into a capillary.

Aseptic technique.
Free from septic matter. Sterile technique.

Autosomal dominant.
Paired chromosomes exerting a ruling influence; dominant trait.

Autosomal recessive.   Paired chromosomes incapable of exerting a ruling or controlling influence unless the respon sible trait is carried by both members of the pair of homologous chromosomes.

Beta-blocker.   Any class of heart drugs that combine with and block the activity of a beta-receptor.

Bio-engineered.   Application to medical science of engineering principles or engineering equipment (construction of artificial heart).

Blood borne pathogens.   Any disease-producing microorganism carried by blood.

Bruit.   The human pulse.

BUN
(Blood Urea Nitrogen).   Urea concentration in the blood or serum stated in terms of nitrogen content.

Cadaver donor.   A person who has died and whose organs are donated for transplantation.

Calcitriol.   The active form of Vitamin D. A preparation of this compound is used to treat hypocalcemia, hypophosphatemia, rickets, and osteodystrophy and other disorders such as renal failure and hypoparathyroidism.

CAT scan *(Computer Axial Tomography).*   The recording of internal body images at a predetermined plane by means of the tomograph.

Catheter.   A flexible tube inserted into a body cavity to withdraw or introduce fluid.

CBC.   Complete blood count.

Cerebrovascular accident/ Cerebrovascular event.   Stroke. A sudden, unexpected interference of blood supply to the brain.

Cerebrovascular event.   An unforeseen occurrence or complicating event of an unfortunate nature involving the blood vessels of the brain, in the course of a disease, or following surgery.

Chloride.   A mineral supplement used in the treatment of copper deficiency.

Creatinine.   The end product of creatine metabolism. Creatine is released into the blood stream during the aerobic phase of muscle contraction, e.g., aerobic exercise.

CMV.   Cytomegalovirus.

Coagulation.   The process of clotting.

Crossmatch.   A blood test to determine the compatibility of donor and recipient.

C&S *(Culture and Sensitivity).*   A mass of microorganisms growing in laboratory culture media. Laboratory method of determining the susceptibility of the patient's bacterial infection to antibiotics.

Cysts.   Any closed cavity or sac, normal or abnormal, lined by epithelium, and especially one that contains a liquid or semisolid material.

Cystogram.   An x-ray of the bladder.

Cystoscopy.   Examination of a bladder with a cystoscope.

Dialysate.   The material that passes through the membrane in dialysis.

Dialysis.   The process of separating crystalloids and colloids in solution. This involved the two processes diffusion and ultrafiltration.

Diffusion.   The movement of solutes (dissolvable substances) across semipermeable membranes.

Diuretic.   An agent which promotes the excretion of urine.

Dry weight.   Estimated "ideal weight." (if estimated dry weight is 110 and the patient weighs in at 115, hemodialysis must remove 5 pounds to achieve 110 pounds when treatment is over).

EBV.   Epstein-Barr Virus. A herpes-like virus which is thought to cause mononucleosis.

ECG *(Electrocardiogram).* A graphic tracing of the variations in electrical potential caused by the excitation of the heart muscle and detected at the body surface.

Edema.   The presence of abnormally large amounts of fluid in the intercellular tissue spaces of the body. Swelling.

Electrolyte.   A substance that disassociates into ions when fused or in solution, and thus becomes capable of conducting electricity.

Embolism. Embolus.   Obstruction of a blood vessel by foreign substances or a blood clot.

Epidural.   Situated upon or outside the dura mater. Injection of an anesthetic directly into the spine.

Epithelium.   The covering of external and internal surfaces of the body including the lining of vessels and other small cavities.

Erythropoietin.   A glycoprotein hormone secreted by the kidneys
Epogen®.   in the adult and by the liver in the fetus, which acts on the bone marrow cells to stimulate red blood cell production.

ESRD.   End-stage renal disease.

Fistula.   An abnormal passage or communication, usually between two internal organs, or leading from an internal organ to the surface of the body.

Graft.   Any tissue, organ or synthetic implement, e.g., prosthesis, for implantation or transplantation.

Hematocrit.   A tube with graduated markings used to determmine the volume of packed red cells in a blood specimen by centrifugation.

Hemodialysis.	The removal of certain elements from the blood by virtue of the rates of their diffusion through a semipermeable membrane.
Hemoglobin.	The oxygen-carrying pigment of the erythrocytes, formed by the developing erythrocyte in the bone marrow.
HLA *(Human Leukocyte Antigen)* typing.	Histocompatibility antigens governed by genes of the HLA complex (the human major histocompatibility complex).
Hypotension.	Abnormally low blood pressure.
Immunosuppressant.	An agent capable of suppressing the immune response.
Inherent. Inherited. Implanted by nature; intrinsic; innate.	The acquisition of characters or qualities by transmission from parent to offspring.
INR *(International Normalization Ratio normal 2.5-3.5).*	The standard used when a patient is maintained on anticoagulation therapy.
Intubate.	The insertion of a tube into a body canal or hollow organ, as into the trachea or stomach.
Living related donor:	A person who is living and who donates an organ to a family member.
Lymphocele.	A sac or pocket containing a collection of fluid.
Lymphocyte.	Any of the mononuclear nonphagocytic leukocytes, found in the blood, lymph, and lymphoid tissues, that are the body's immunologically competent cells and their precursors.
MRI *(Magnetic resonance imaging).*	A type of x-ray which produces a three-dimensional view of a body part.
Nephrology. Nephrologist.	Scientific study of the kidney, its anatomy, physiology, pathology and pathophysiology.

Palpate. Palpation.   To examine using the hands.

PICC-line *(Peripherally*   A catheter usually inserted in the inner, upper
                                  ams.

Inserted Central Catheter). There are two ports, one for blood drawing and
                                  the other for infusing medications.

PKD *(Polycystic Kidney*   Hereditary kidney disease causing many cysts in
Disease).   the kidneys.

Pathology.   That branch of medicine which deals with the
                  structural and functional changes in tissues and
                  organs of the body caused by disease.

Peritonitis.   Inflammation of the peritoneum, the membranous
                    coat lining the abdominal cavity and invading the
                    viscera.

Phosphorus.   A nonmetallic allotropic element, poisonous and
                   highly inflammable; occurring in bones, urine
                   and especially in minerals such as apatite. Very
                   essential in the diet. The major component in
                   bones and essential in all metabolic processes.

Platelets.   Round or oval discs measuring approximately 2-4
                  micra, numbering 200,000/300,000 cu. mm.
                  They contain no hemoglobin and play an impor-
                  tant role in blood coagulation, hemostasis, and
                  blood thrombus formation.

Potassium.   An electrolyte administered orally or via IV.

TED® **hose.**   Very snug fitting elastic stockings used by
                      patients during major surgery to minimize the
                      risk of blood clots in the legs.

PT *(Prothrombin Time).*   Substance in the blood essential to the clotting
                                process hence, to the maintenance of normal
                                hemostasis. Normal range is (11.6-14.7 seconds).

PTT *(Partial*   Clotting time. A substance having procoagulant
Thromboplastin Time).   properties or activity. Normal range (22.7-36.1
                           seconds).

Pulse. Pulsatile. The rhythmic expansion of an artery which may be felt with the finger.

Reflux. A backward flow.

Rejection. An immune response against grafted tissue that may result in failure of the graft to survive.

Sedative. An agent that allays activity and excitement.

Sensitized. Sensitization. A condition of being made sensitive to a specific substance (e.g. antigen) such as a protein.

Septic. Sepsis. Putrefying or pathogenic organisms or their toxins.

Spinal tap. Procedure whereby a long needle is inserted into the spine for the purpose of removing spinal fluid for analysis or introducing medication.

Staphylococcus aureus. A species of bacteria commonly present on skin and mucous membranes, especially nose and mouth. A cause of suppurative conditions such as boils, caruncles and abscesses.

Thrill. A sensation of vibration felt by the examiner on palpation of the body, as over the heart during loud, harsh cardiac murmurs.

Thrombosis. Thrombus. The formation or development of a blood clot or thrombus. It is a solid aggregation formed in circulating blood and such changes constitute thrombosis.

TIA *(Transient Ischemic Attack).* Stroke-like symptoms of short duration generally produced by an insufficient oxygen supply to the brain. Clots are the general cause.

Titer. Standard of strength per volume of volumetric test solution.

Toxin. A poisonous substance of animal or plant origin.

Transfusion. The introduction of whole blood or blood component directly into the blood stream.

Tubules.	A small tube.
Tumor.	Swelling, one of the cardinal signs of inflammation; a new growth of tissue in which the multiplication of cells is uncontrolled and progressive.
UA *(Urinalysis).*	Analysis of the urine.
Ultrafiltration.	Filtration through filters with minute pores, thus allowing the separation of extremely minute particles.
Ultrasound *(ultrasonogram).*	The visualization of deep structures in the body by recording the reflections of (echoes of) pulses of ultrasonic waves directed into the tissues.
Ureters.	Tubes carrying urine from the kidneys to the bladder.
Vessel.	A tube, duct, or canal to convey the body's fluids.
Vital signs.	Blood pressure, pulse, respiration and temperature.
VCU (Voiding Cystourethrogram).	A test performed to determine to what extent the urinary ladder is emptying.
Yeast.	Any of several unicellular fungi which reproduce by budding.

APPENDIX - A
POLYCYSTIC KIDNEY DISEASE

PKD occurs throughout the world and does not discriminate between socio-economic or ethnic groups. Men and women are affected equally. About 12.5 million people world wide are affected by PKD. About 600,000 Americans alone are affected by PKD, making it two times more common than multiple sclerosis and 20 times more common than cystic fibrosis.

Although PKD is the most common life-threatening genetic disease, few people know of its existence. The Polycystic Kidney Research Foundation is the only organization worldwide solely devoted to promoting programs of research into the cause, treatment and cure of PKD. The PKD Foundation is not a United Way Agency and receives no federal or state funding. Lyme disease receives $62 million in federal research funds although it is 45 times less prevalent than PKD and can be readily treated with a vaccination which has recently become available. The Polycystic Kidney Research Foundation provides any levels of membership and contributions to the PKR Foundation are tax deductible. For further information contact:

The Polycystic Kidney Research Foundation
4901 Main Street, Suite 20
Kansas City, MO 64112-2634
1-816-931-8655 or 1-800-PKD-CURE

PKD affects both kidneys causing them to enlarge. The symptoms include: back pain, blood in the urine (caused by blood vessels breaking in the cysts), kidney stones, and recurring bladder or kidney infections and high blood pressure, which occurs in 60 percent of PKD patients.

Complications of the disease include: loss of kidney function, brain aneurysms, mitral valve prolapse in the heart, frequent infections, chronic flank or back pain, pancreas or liver cysts, enlarged heart, kidney stones, groin or abdominal hernias, and diverticulitis of the colon. A high percentage of patients with PKD develop kidney failure, requiring dialysis treatments or a kidney transplant to maintain their life. Symptoms of kidney failure emerge when five to ten percent of kidney function remains.

For this reason, 40% of the people with the disease are unaware that they have it. These symptoms include: loss of appetite, nausea, vomiting, fatigue, itching, and muscle twitching. If untreated, the buildup of waste products become toxic and will lead to coma, seizures, and death.

PKD is diagnosed by taking either x-rays, ultrasonograms or CAT scans. Of the three, the CAT scan is the most sensitive because of the use of contrast (dye).

LEFT - POLYCYSTIC KIDNEY / RIGHT - NORMAL KIDNEY

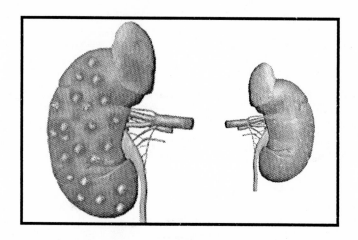

There is no specific treatment for PKD. Patients with PKD should be closely monitored. Current options include managing the disease through careful control of high blood pressure, prompt treatment for kidney or bladder infections, adherence to a protein restricted diet to decrease the rate of kidney function loss, and exercise to maintain good physical condition.

Patients with PKD very seldom have the energy or stamina required to participate in a regular exercise regimen. For this reason, the exercises recommended include: walking, swimming and bicycling. Contact sports should be avoided since patients with enlarged kidneys may have increased chance of bleeding. Abstaining from contact sports is also recommended for patients on Coumadin® (anticoagulant) therapy.

Pregnancy is fairly safe for women with PKD who have normal kidney function and have only minor symptoms of the disease. The risk to the mother is increased if she is hypertensive, and the likelihood of carrying the pregnancy to term is reduced.

Research has located the abnormal gene for PKD on chromosome 14. Currently, there are tests available to detect this gene. Research is also underway to determine if chemicals can be developed to treat the cysts which grow as benign tumors, and if the use of diuretics (water pills) can be used to prevent the build-up of fluid in the cysts.

APPENDIX - B
LIST OF PHOSPHORUS-RICH FOODS

Bananas
Melons (Watermelon, Cantaloupe, Honeydew)
Self-rising flour
Baking powder
Baked goods (pancakes, waffles, doughnuts, cookies)
Raw bran (unprocessed)
Bran products (muffins, cereal, bread, etc)

Malted milks
Milk shakes
Instant milk drink mixed
Yogurt
Cheese, spreads or cheese products
Ice cream
Malts
Sherbet
Puddings, custards
Eggnog

Legumes, dried peas and beans
Frozen, canned and fresh peas or beans
Baked beans
Nuts, peanut butter
Seeds, sunflower, pumpkin, etc.
Granola
Dark breads, breads with seeds or nuts
Corn bread, corn dogs
Potato chips, tortilla chips, cheese snacks or crackers

Limit fish to no more than 2 ounces per serving
Sardines
Liver and organ meats

Avocados
Dried fruit
Chocolate, cocoa
Cola beverages
Beer
Molasses

CARE OF A FISTULA AND FISTULA ARM

* Never wear tight fitting clothing on the arm because this could obstruct blood flow and cause a clot.
* Avoid injury to the arm.
* Never sleep on the arm; this could cause clotting.
* Wash fistula gently with soap and water while bathing. Rubbing vigorously could dislodge a clot.
* Do not allow blood drawing, the taking of blood pressures, or the placement of IVs on the fistula arm.
* During winter months keep fistula arm warm to avoid aching.
* Check fistula every day for a pulse which feels like a buzz. If you cannot feel the buzz, contact your nephrologist immediately. Also, check for redness or drainage, which are signs of infection.
* Do not lift heavy objects.

After dialysis I was advised to:

* Remove outer gauze dressing before going to bed.
* Check over access site for signs of a bruit or buzz.
* Remove the adhesive bandages the following day after dialysis.
* Should bleeding occur, apply direct pressure over the bleeding area with fingers of your other hand.
* If bleeding exceeds ten minutes notify nephrologist or vascular surgeon and go to the Emergency Room.
* If needle accidentally punctures the side of your access apply ice for 24 hours to reduce the infiltration or swelling. If swelling increases, notify your nephrologist. Apply moist heat the following day for 24 hours and as always check over access site for signs of a bruit or buzz. If there is no bruit or buzz, notify your nephrologist or vascular surgeon immediately.

APPENDIX - D
PERITONEAL DIALYSIS (PD)

An access for peritoneal dialysis is surgically placed in the lower abdomen, just below the navel and to one side. It tunnels through the fat and muscle tissue then enters the peritoneal cavity. The end of the catheter lies on the floor of the peritoneal cavity. A portion of the catheter (2 to 6 inches) is left outside the body for easy connection to the dialysis tubing. The access has two cuffs that are placed in this tunnel. These cuffs help the tissue grow around the catheter so that it cannot easily be removed. Cleaning solution called dialysate travels through the access into the abdomen.

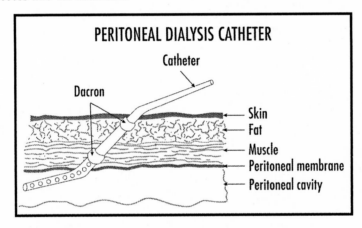

Peritoneal dialysis does the same work as hemodialysis, which is to replace the work of the kidneys. This type of dialysis however, uses the lining of the abdomen to filter the blood through the principles of osmosis and diffusion. This lining is called the peritoneal membrane. The peritoneal membrane is filled with little tiny blood vessels.

Because of kidney failure, the blood contains an excess amount of fluid, chemicals and wastes. Through the principles of osmosis and diffusion, the excess fluid, chemicals, and wastes leave the blood vessels, cross the peritoneal membrane and enter the dialysate. When both the blood and the dialysate have equal amounts of fluid, chemicals and wastes, dialysis stops.

The dialysate must be drained from the peritoneal cavity and replaced with fresh dialysate. CAPD requires that the patient dialyze continuously, denying the fluid, chemicals, and waste the opportunity to increase to an unacceptable level in the blood. Dialysate actually stays in the peritoneal cavity at all times, except, during draining and replacing the dialysate. The dialysate is replaced several times every day. In my particular case five times per day.

The pros of PD as I see them include:

1. A smaller catheter which stays in place through a small hole in the abdomen made by a surgeon.

2. I do not have to be stuck with needles.

3. I do not have to worry about having to apply pressure for 15-20 minutes at the treatment site on completion of treatment.

4. There is no concern about clotting accesses since blood would not be involved.

5. No highs before and lows after treatment because PD is a slow and gradual process.

6. I can lead a very normal life.

7. I can use bath gels and body washes instead of cake soaps because cake soaps retain bacteria and could potentially infect my access site.

8. I also enjoy the freedom of not being tied to a machine for 3 hours, 3 times a week.

9. Peritoneal dialysis gives me an element of control in an otherwise uncontrollable situation. I perform my own treatments at home and at work.

10. My diet is not as stringent as with hemodialysis. In fact, PD requires the consumption of more protein, salt, and fruit for potassium because of the loss of electrolytes (sodium, potassium, chloride and CO_2) during the PD process.

11. The time it takes me to perform the entire treatment starting with washing my hands, draining and re-filling, then washing my hands again, takes approximately 30 minutes.

12. If I intend to travel, I would let my supply company know in what state or country I plan to vacation. They will arrange to deliver my supplies where I'll be staying, a week before I arrive.

The cons of PD as I see them include:

1. I need to be well disciplined because I am in charge of my treatments.

2. No hot-tubing, swimming in lakes, or baths because of the risk of infection entering through my access site. I can swim in pools but my access site dressing has to be changed immediately after exiting the pool. Sitting in a wet swimsuit is also discouraged.

3. The room in which I would perform my PD must be scrupulously clean and dust free. No pets are allowed in the room. No one else is allowed in the room with me unless they are wearing a mask.

4. The heating or air conditioning must not be active while I am performing my treatment, to avoid the circulation of dust particles or bacteria.

5. All PD patients from time to time are afflicted with bouts of peritonitis, some more frequently than others. This can be avoided by using proper aseptic technique and keeping my surroundings clean.

6. Exit site dressing has to be changed after every shower.

7. I can no longer wear tight clothing (e.g. tight jeans) because they cause discomfort, also, I now have an access to conceal.

8. I do require a substantial amount of room to store my PD supplies, e.g., a month's worth of supplies for me consists of approximately 42 boxes.

9. During menstruation, the dialysate drained from my peritoneal cavity is pink to red, and draining and filling is sometimes a bit uncomfortable.

10. For some patients, the access site never heals. This happens because the catheter moves slightly in and out at the access exit site.

APPENDIX - E
ADVANCE MEDICAL DIRECTIVES
LIVING WILL DECLARATION

An Advance Directive protects people during extreme conditions such as irreversible brain damage, permanent coma or terminal illness. Advance Directive can limit life-prolonging measures such as cardiopulmonary resuscitation (CPR), IV therapy, feeding tubes, respirators and dialysis. Provision is also made for pain relief and organ donation if desired.

A Living Will is a document which stipulates the kind of life-prolonging care you want if you become terminally ill and unable to make your own decisions. A Durable Power of Attorney names a person or (proxy) who makes decision for you if you become incapacitated. Let your values and religion be your guide when making this caliber of decision. Advance Directives can be changed or revoked at any time.

* Check the laws in your state.
* Put your wishes in writing. Sign, date, and have your
  Advance Directive witnessed by two people who are
  not your spouse or blood relative (or an adopted relative).
* Keep a card in your wallet stating that you have an
  Advance Directive.
* Give your physician a copy for your medical record.
* Discuss your Advance Directive with your family,
  physician, clergy member and attorney.

It is important to note that there is no cost to the donor family or estate for any organs or tissues donated. All expenses associated with recovery procedures become the responsibility of the recovering organization. Expenses associated with hospitalization prior to the donation, funeral and burial arrangements remain the responsibility of the family or estate.

For further information or for a free copy of a living will or durable power of attorney contact a hospital, lawyer, State Attorney General's Office or:

The Society for the Right to Die/ Choice in Dying,
250 West 57th Street, New York, NY 10107.
1-212-246-6973.

This organization will provide copies of living-will forms free of charge.

APPENDIX - F
SEX POST TRANSPLANTATION

Many post transplant patients experience difficulties relative to sex and intimacy. The transplant is usually named as the culprit when problems of this nature are experienced. In actuality, fatigue, depression, unreal expectations, poor body image, or dissatisfaction with a partner are in fact the culprits.

This is not an easy subject for most people to discuss. When the subject of sex is broached, even health care professionals can become uncomfortable. Sex is a quality-of-life issue and must be dealt with. Many patients are ready to return to an active sex life while yet others are afraid of such intimacy because of their scars and weight gain. There is a fear of not being attractive anymore. Excessive hair growth as a result of steroid use causes many patients to experience poor self image. Some blame their spouse's reluctance to participate in sexual activity on their scars and weight gain. A great majority of the time, the spouse's reluctance to participate in sexual activity is due to their fear of causing pain or discomfort to the recently transplanted patient. This, to me, would seem to be a communication issue. Take heart, the excessive hair growth can be removed, and the weight gain can be corrected through diet and exercise.

People are not comfortable revealing what their wants or desires are to their partner for fear of rejection or ridicule. The transplant patient must find a way to discuss the subject of sex with their partner. If not discussed the matter can never be resolved. This could lead to resentment, which causes stress, and in turn leads to sexual tension.

In yet other cases, the problem may be medication induced. For example, blood pressure medications and steroids may cause a decrease in sexual desire or impotency. Because of immunosuppression, the transplant patient should not use anything with oil, sugar or flavoring, as these may cause yeast infections. In some cases the problems and fears experienced by transplant patients go beyond the mere physical. In my opinion, a serious discussion with a health care professional is recommended, because these patients may require antidepressants or psychological counseling.

GUIDELINES FOR WRITING
TO DONOR FAMILIES

A topic that is often thought about, but not often brought up for conversation is one of the donor family. Up to this point the focus has been on the physical aspect of the transplant, learning your new medications and dosages, dealing with side effects of the new drugs, and waiting for your incision to heal. During your quiet times, I'm sure your thoughts go to your donor family. Organ donation is such a wonderful gift, and it is hard to believe that such a wonderful gift could generate at the same time so much sadness because of the loss of someone's life. Many times a recipient will find some closure regarding their donor by writing the donor family to thank them for their new lease on life. In turn you will be bringing some closure to the donor family, who gave unselfishly so others could have a second change in life. Writing this letter is not an easy task, and we hope that by giving you some guidelines to follow, it will make it easier. You may send a letter or greeting card.

Talking about yourself:
* Use your first name only.
* Use the State in which you live (not the city).
* Talk about your family situation. (Marital status, children, grandchildren, dogs, cats, birds. Use first names only).
* Talk about your hobbies.
* You may talk about your religious beliefs.

Talking about your Transplant Experience:
* Describe how long you waited for a transplant and what was the wait like for you and your family.
* Explain how the transplant has changed or improved your life.
* Talk about experiences that have happened since your transplant, such as birthdays, trips, outings, possibly a new job!
* Recognize the donor family and thank them for their gift.

Closing your letter or card:
* Sign your first name only.
* Do not reveal your address, city, phone number or location of your hospital or physician.

Mail or take your letter to your transplant coordinator

URINARY TRACT INFECTIONS (UTI's)

UTI's occur when bacteria enter through the urethra and travel to the bladder and/or kidneys. Most often these infections are caused by Escherichia coli, which usually occurs in the intestines. Another cause of infections occur because of a blockage of the normal flow of urine, precipitated by an obstruction such as an enlarged prostate gland, kidney stone or other abnormality of the urinary tract.

Women are much more susceptible to UTI's due to the fact that a woman's urethra is much shorter than a man's and bacteria have a much shorter distance to travel. Some women are susceptible to UTI's through sexual intercourse. After menopause, UTI's may increase because of a lack of certain hormones. UTIs also seem to be precipitated by a woman's method of birth control. Studies have shown that women who use a diaphragm are more likely to have a UTI than women who use other methods of birth control.

To following steps can be taken to reduce the risk of contracting a UTI:

* Do not postpone urinating when you feel the urge.
* Do not rush, take the time when you urinate to empty your
  bladder completely.
* Respond to your body's signals of thirst by drinking enough
  water or other liquids every day.
* Urinate after sexual intercourse.
* Wipe genital area from front to back.

THE MENTOR PROGRAM
TRIO HOTLINE MENTORS

Apart from the MENTOR program, good sources of information are doctors, transplant coordinators, nurses or social workers, but they all possess one big drawback, they are not transplant recipients. They can provide the clinical information but they do not fully understand the changes we are forced to go through, or what the medications do to our minds and bodies. This is another example of the benefit of the MENTOR program, which provides someone to talk to who understands exactly what we as transplant patients are going through.

The San Diego Transplant Association Mentor Program is a peer fellowship program for patients and family members going through the transplant process, pre- or post-transplant. It provides specific training for their mentors in the clinical and interpersonal skills areas. They are also trained to look and listen for signs of anger, hopelessness, denying the need for transplantation, or refusing their life saving dialysis treatments. The MENTOR program also attempts to match patient and mentor on the basis of similarities of their problems.

Starting a MENTOR program requires the involvement of the local transplant staff and approval of transplant program administrators. SDTA representatives or trainers are sent to the city in question to provide the specific training needed to administer the program correctly. Volunteers expenses and an honorarium to the SDTA treasury is required for the Copyrighted materials and training. In the past, MENTOR programs have been sponsored by pharmaceutical companies or grants. Funding is also available through the Transplant Programs in your area. For further information contact Shawn Faulk at 1-619-687-0245.

(TRIO) The Transplant Recipients International Organization provides "Hot Line Mentors" whose role is to:

* Be a good listener and respect patient's confidentiality
* Share their experiences and provide reassurance
* Serve as compliment to medical staff
* Log contacts with patient's and maintain progress notes
* Be alert to areas needing extra support and refer to appropriate support services
* Referral to sources for life-changing problems relating to transplantation

To qualify as a "Hot Line Mentor:"

*   You must be one year post transplantation and compliant
    with your transplant center's program
*   Must have a positive attitude and healthy perspective
*   Must have a realistic view of transplantation
*   Must be committed to the program concept
*   Must be willing to sign a confidentiality statement

APPENDIX - J
TOTAL HIP REPLACEMENT

A total hip replacement is performed by cutting the ball from the thigh bone. The damaged ball is replaced with a metal ball and a metal stem which is fitted into the femur. The surface of the old socket is smoothed then a new plastic socket is implanted into the pelvis, replacing the damaged socket. Among the types of metals used are: stainless steel, alloys of cobalt and chrome, and titanium. The plastic material (polyethylene) is durable and wear resistant. Currently, orthopaedic surgeons can replace, hips, knees, ankles, feet, shoulders, elbows, and finger joints.

The possible risks and complications to total hip replacement are: reaction to anesthesia, blood clots, infection, dislocation of the joint, damage to surrounding blood vessels, bones and nerves, and thigh pain. The benefits to hip replacement are: reduction in hip pain, increased leg and muscle strength, improved quality of life, and ease of movement. There is a certain amount of post surgical pain initially because of inactivity and healing of the muscles surrounding the joint. The pain however, will abate after a few weeks. The majority of patients stand and walk the day after surgery.

To make your recovery period more comfortable certain preparations should be made at home, these are: store frequently used items at waist level, stock up on canned foods, prepare a room on the main living level if your bedroom is upstairs, pick up clutter, remove throw rugs and tape down electrical cords. Special equipment required include: an elevated toilet seat, a shower seat, a walker, a cane, and a grasping device for pulling on socks and shoes.

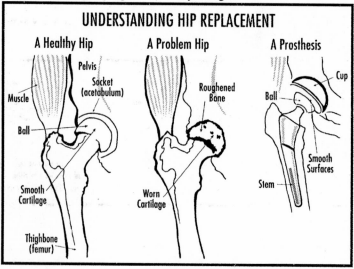

140

APPENDIX - K
CATARACTS

It is believed that cataracts are associated with smoking, diabetes, changes in age, certain vitamins and minerals. Some health care providers believe that simply taking certain vitamins and minerals may prevent or delay the formation of cataracts.

The symptoms experienced by patients with cataracts include: cloudy or blurred vision, sensitivity to light, especially automobile headlights at night, which appear to have a halo around them, colors appear faded, double vision, and frequent changes in contact lenses or eyeglasses.

Cataracts grow slowly, therefore, impairment of vision is gradual. Cataracts come in different types; they are: age-related cataracts, the most common type, congenital cataracts, meaning babies are born with them, secondary cataracts, due to a health problem (diabetes) or medication induced (steroids), and traumatic cataracts, which may develop after an eye injury.

Cataracts have to be removed when the degree of impairment begins to affect the patient's quality of life. Cataract surgery is performed on only one eye at a time, and patient's having this surgery experience much better vision afterwards. This type of surgery is currently being performed on an outpatient basis, and patient's go home the same day. On rare occasions, there is some bleeding, and the patient is admitted for observation.

After surgery patient's may experience itchy or sticky eyelids and some mild discomfort. The healing process usually takes approximately six weeks. Immediately after surgery, a patient is able to read or watch television.

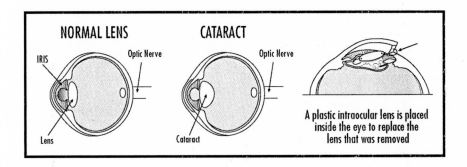

A plastic intraocular lens is placed
inside the eye to replace the
lens that was removed

MULTIPLE DRUG RESISTANT (MDR) BACTERIA & CONTACT ISOLATION

MDR bacteria are bacteria which are extremely difficult to destroy with anti-biotics. People who are likely to contract an MDR bacteria are: those who have had many antibiotics, weakened immune systems, chronically ill or who have had prolonged hospital stays. A person may have this type of MDR bacteria present and not be ill. These bacteria are present in urine, blood, stool, wounds, and other body fluids. These MDR bacteria are treated with specialized antibiotics via IV.

Sometimes when patients are taken off antibiotics or achieve a better degree of health, their bodies can destroy these bacteria by themselves.

These MDR bacteria are highly infectious and to avoid the spread of such bacteria a patient in the hospital will be placed on Contact Isolation. Gowns, masks and gloves must be worn by everyone entering the patient's room. This includes health care providers, family and friends alike. Gowns and gloves are disposed of before leaving the patient's room. Hand washing with antiseptic soap and the disposal of masks are both observed after leaving the patient's room.

MDR bacteria can live on surfaces for a period of several days, therefore, any equipment used in the patient's room must remain in the room. When on Contact Isolation a patient is required to stay in their rooms unless specifically directed to do otherwise.

ORGANIZATIONS THAT CAN HELP

American Kidney Fund
Suite 1010
6110 Executive Boulevard
Rockville, MD 20852 1-800-638-8299

American Association of Kidney Patients
Suite LL1
1 Davis Boulevard
Tampa, FL 33606 1-813-251-0725

National Kidney Foundation, Inc.
30 East 33rd Street
New York, NY 10016 800-622-9010

National Kidney Foundation
Northeast Florida Division
80 West Eighth Street
Jacksonville, FL 32209 904-366-7913

National Kidney and Urology Diseases
Information Clearinghouse
Box NKUDIC
9000 Rockville Pike
Bethesda, MD 20892 301-654-4415

The Sandoz Transplant Learning Center
Do not tough it out alone. A team of physicians to answer all your
questions, providing understanding and encouragement. For more
information or to enroll call 888-852-3683

Best Care Transplant Pharmacy Program
Sponsored by Stadtlanders Pharmacy *(Experts in transplant
pharmaceutical care)* To enroll in this program write to:
SDC
Attn: Enrollment
600 Penn Center Blvd.
Pittsburgh, PA 15235-9928
800-238-7828 E-mail: www.stadtlander.com

UNINSURED HOTLINE

The Florida Comprehensive Health Association (FCHA)
Uninsurable Hotline for Floridians who are able to obtain Private Health Insurance
1-888-676-3242

SHINE - Serving Health Insurance Needs of Elders
(provides free health insurance counseling for elders)
Florida Department of Elder Affairs
SHINE PROGRAM
1317 Winewood Blvd., E
Room 430
Tallahassee, FL 32399-0700

MEDICARE HANDBOOK
U.S. Government Printing Office
U.S. Department of Health and Human Services
Health Care Financing Administration
7500 Security Boulevard
Baltimore, Maryland 21244-1850

Medicare Coverage of Kidney Dialysis and Kidney Transplant Services
(A supplement to your Medicare Handbook)
U.S. Department of Health and Human Services
6325 Security Boulevard
Baltimore, Maryland 21207-5187

DONATE YOUR USED CAR
TO THE NATIONAL KIDNEY FOUNDATION

*   Help drive down the rate of kidney disease while saving the environment.

*   Donate your used car. You may qualify for a tax deduction.

For further information call: 1(800)488-CARS (2277).

Calling this **NATIONWIDE TELEPHONE NUMBER** will activate a chain of events.

The National Kidney Foundation will telephone a local towing company in your area and make all arrangements for the free pick-up and delivery of your donated used car to the participating organization or your local National Kidney Foundation.

End Stage Renal Disease Network of Florida, Inc.
Florida ESRD Patient Services Committee
1 Davis Blvd., Suite 304
Tampa, FL 33606

DIALYSIS CENTERS

Dialysis Centers, Inc.
4221 Southpoint Blvd.,
Jacksonville, FL 32216
904-296-6362

Dialysis Centers, Inc.
615-617 Park Street
Jacksonville, FL 32204
904-355-6602

Baptist Medical Center
800 Prudential Drive
Jacksonville, FL 32207
904-390-1684

FMC dba/Jacksonville Kidney Center
3132 St. John's Bluff
Jacksonville, FL 32246
904-641-0806

FMC dba/Jacksonville Kidney Center
1107 Myra Street, Ste. 101
Jacksonville, FL 32204
904-354-3333

FMC dba/Jacksonville Kidney Center
1715 Kings Avenue
Jacksonville, FL 32207
904-396-7203

FMC North Jacksonville
10614 Lem Turner Road
Jacksonville, FL 32218
904-768-8576

FMC dba/Renal Care Centers
201 Health Park Blvd.,
St. Augustine, FL 32084
904-824-6191

Human Resources Group
1525 Lime Street, Ste. 120
Fernandina Beach, FL 32034
904-491-1998

Jupiter Kidney Center
1000 Old Dixie Hwy.
Jupiter, FL 33458
407-744-4661

North East Florida Dialysis
2020 Kingsley Avenue, Ste. B
Orange Park, FL 32073
904-272-7331

North Palm Beach Dialysis
3375 Burns Road, Ste. 101
Palm Beach, FL 33410
407-775-8700

Methodist Med. Ctr. Dialysis
580 West Eighth Street
Jacksonville, FL 32207
904-366-7903

Shands/Methodist Med. Ctr.
655 West Eighth Street
Jacksonville, FL 32207
Hemo-904-549-6690
Peritoneal-904-549-4370

Shands/University Med. Ctr.
655 West Eighth Street
Jacksonville, FL 32206
904-350-6899 Ext. 4516

St. Augustine Kidney Center
264 South Park Circle E.
St. Augustine, FL 32086
904-808-0445

The Dialysis at Sea Traveller Cruises, 801 West Bay Dr.,
Ste. 800, Largo, FL 33770 800-544-7604

Each patient's center is determined by their insurance company.

APPENDIX - Q
FINANCIAL ASSISTANCE

American Organ Transplant Association (AOTA)
P.O. Box 277
Stafford, TX 77459 281-261-2682
(Provides transportation to/from centers and accommodation; administers transplant trust fund)

American Liver Foundation
1425 Pompton Avenue
Cedar Grove, NJ 07009 800-366-2682
(Provides fund-raising information)

Children's Organ Transplant Association (COTA)
2501 Cota Drive
Bloomington, IN 47403 800-366-2682
(Assists with fund-raising events; direct financial assistance)

National Organization for Rare Diseases (NORD)
Medical Assistance Program
P.O. Box 823
New Fairfield, CT 06812-1783 800-447-NORD
(Helps supply free Sandimmune to qualified patients.)

Organ Transplant Fund, Inc.
P.O. Box 41903
Memphis, TN 38174
(Organizes fund-raisers; tax-deductible donations can be made on a patient's behalf)

The National Heart Association and Transplant Fund
519 W. Lancaster Avenue
Hartford, PA 19401 800-642-8399
(Non-profit group providing financial, social and emotional support)

Transplant Foundation
8002 Discovery Drive
Suite 310
Richmond, VA 23229
804-285-5115
(Arranges short-term post transplant medication assistance)

The List, Dialysis & Transplantation Magazine
Released every July
(provides an international listing of dialysis centers accepting visitors, on vacation or business travel) Book well in advance of travel; Medicare pays 80 percent of the cost 800-442-5667

The National Listing of Medicare Providers Furnishing Kidney Dialysis and Transplant Services 202-512-1800

MENTOR PROGRAM (Jacksonville, FL)
(TRIO) Transplant Recipients International Organization
Held once a month at St. Vincent's Hospital
    1800 Barrs Street
    Jacksonville, FL 32204
    904-308-7300

MENTOR PROGRAM (Nationwide)
San Diego Transplant Association **(SDTA)** For location of program near you and for information on how to start a MENTOR program in your area contact:
    J. Shawn Faulk, MS, RD, CDE
    SDTA President
    619-437-6766

TRANSPLANT DRUG PROGRAMS

CHRONIMED - 800-888-5753
Continental Health Care - 900-776-4633
CURA Script Pharmacy - 888-773-7376
Good Life Resources, Inc. - 800-227-2111
Mayo Clinic Comprehensive Drug Therapy Program - 800-337-3736
Statlanders Pharmacy - 800-238-7828

RESOURCE CENTERS AND SUPPORT GROUPS

American Association of Kidney Patients (AAKP)
111 South Parker Street
Suite 405
Tampa, FL 33606
800-749-2257
*(**Nationwide** support group for transplant patients and their families)*

Transplant Recipient International Organization (TRIO)
244 N. Bellfield Avenue
Pittsburgh, PA 15213
412-687-2210
*(**Nationwide** support group for transplant patients and their families)*

Bone Marrow Transplant Support Network
(800)826-9376
*(**Nationwide** support network for Bone Marrow Transplant patients and their families)*

National Kidney Foundation, Inc.
30 East 33rd Street
New York, NY 10016
800-622-9010
> *Provides the following brochures:*
> * Working with Kidney Disease
>   *(**Rehabilitation and Employment**)*
> * Coping Effectively
>   *(**A guide for patients and their families**)*
> * Urinary Tract Infections
> * Polycystic Kidney Disease
> * Peritoneal Dialysis-An Alternative to Hemodialysis
> * Sexuality and Chronic Kidney Disease

On the Road Again
*(**A Nationwide Travel Guide for Dialysis Patients**)*
NMC Patient Travel Service
A Free Service
800-634-6254

ADDITIONAL SOURCES OF INFORMATION

Your New Life With Dialysis - A Patient Guide for Physical and Psychological Adjustments
Edith T. Oberley, M.A., and Terry D. Oberley, M.D., Ph.D.
Fourth edition, 1991
    Charles C. Thomas Publishers
    2600 South First Street
    Springfield, IL 62794-9265

Understanding Kidney Transplantation
Edith T. Oberley, M.A., and Neal R. Glass, M.D., F.A.C.S.
    Charles C. Thomas Publishers, 1987
    2600 South First Street
    Springfield, IL 62794-9265

Kidney Disease: A Guide for Patients and Their Families
    American Kidney Fund
    Suite 2020
    6100 Executive Boulevard
    Rockville, MD 20852
    800-638-8299

National Kidney Foundation Patient Education Brochures
Includes information on treatment, diet, work, and exercise.
    National Kidney Foundation, Inc.
    30 East 33rd Street
    New York, NY 10016
    800-622-9010

Medicare Coverage of Kidney Dialysis and Kidney Transplant Services. A Supplement to Your Medicare Handbook
Publication Number HCFA-02183
    U.S. Department of Health and Human Services
    Health Care Financing Administration
    Suite 500
    1331 H. Street, NW
    Washington, DC 20005 301-966-7843

ADDITIONAL SOURCES OF READING/EDUCATION

Renalife Magazine
American Association of Kidney Patients (AAKP)
Suite LL1
1 Davis Boulevard
Tampa, FL 33606
813-251-0725 (Published quarterly)

Family Focus Newsletter
National Kidney Foundation, Inc.
30 East 33rd Street
New York, NY 10016
800-622-9010

Contemporary Dialysis & Nephrology &
For Patients Only Magazine
Suite 400
20335 Ventura Boulevard
Woodland Hills, Ca 91364
818-704-5555 (Published six times per year)

The Partnership for Organ Donation
One International Place
Boston, MA 02110 617-330-8650
(A non-profit organization)

American Heart Association
7272 Greenville Avenue
Dallas, TX 75231
800-AHA-USA1

Transplant Chronicles National Kidney Foundation
30 East 33rd Street
New York, NY 10016

Transdial
Newsletter for Florida Kidney Transplant & Dialysis Patients
Florida Renal Coalition
Patient Services Program
1 Davis Boulevard, Suite 304
Tampa, FL. 33606
813-254-2558 or 800-826-3773

Patient Services
1 Davis Blvd., Suite 304
Tampa, FL 33606 800-826-3773

Kidney News
National Kidney Foundation of Florida, Inc.
1040 Woodcock Road, Suite 119
Orlando, FL 32803

ENCORE
CHRONIMED Publishing
P.O. Box 59032
Minneapolis, MN 55459-9686

Contemporary Dialysis & Nephrology Magazine
Attention: Subscription Department
18 East 41st Street, 20th Floor
New York, NY 10017

The PKR Progress
The Polycystic Kidney Research Foundation
4901 Main Street, Suite 200
Kansas City, MO 64112-2634
800-PKD-CURE FAX: 816-931-8655
e-mail: pkdcure@pkrfoundation.org

*The PKD Foundation provides many books for those who wish to
learn more about PKD:*

* The Family and ADPKD: A Guide for children and Parents
* PKD Patient's Manual (Understanding and Living with polycystic
  kidney disease)
* Q&A on PKD
* Oxford Nephrology Series - Polycystic Kidney Disease
* 2ND EDITION YOUR CHILD, YOUR FAMILY AND
  AUTOSOMAL RECESSIVE POLYCYSTIC KIDNEY DISEASE

PATIENT CONFERENCE/SEMINAR

End Stage Renal Disease Network of Florida, Inc.
The Florida Renal Coalition
Patient Services Program
1 Davis Building, Suite 304
Tampa, FL 33606
800-826-3773
813-254-2558

The Polycystic Kidney Research Foundation
4901 Main Street, Suite 200
Kansas City, MO 64112-2634
816-931-2600 or 800-PKD-CURE
FAX: 816-931-8655
e-mail: pkdcure@pkrfoundation.org

The PKD Research Foundation sponsors many conferences. Contact them at the above numbers for upcoming conferences. Ask the Foundation also to mail you the PKR Progress.

Look for conferences and seminars held in your city or state.

For information on Guided Imagery contact:
Diane Tusek, RN, BSN
Cleveland Clinic Foundation
440-944-9292, fax: 440-944-1830

For further information or to order **Loretta LaRoche's tapes "the Joy of Stress," "How Serious Is This,"**
"Humor Your Stress," contact or call
WGBH Boston Video/Dept. 9913
P.O. Box 2284
South Burlington, VT 05407-2284
800-949-8670 Ext. 9913
802-864-9846 Ext. 9913 (for fax orders)

APPENDIX - V
TESTS AND SYMPTOMS OF
ABNORMAL LEVELS

Alb - Albumin: Method of measuring nutrition.

Alk Phos - Alkaline Phosphatase: Indicative of bone, liver or gallbladder disease. Painful joints and weak bones.

BUN - Blood Urea Nitrogen: Too much protein. Fatigue, nausea, insomnia, dry itching skin, and urine-like body and breath odor.

CA - Calcium: Too much phosphorus-rich foods. Low: Muscle spasms, cramping, seizures, and hair loss. High: Muscle weakness, fatigue, constipation, nausea, vomiting and loss of appetite.

Chol - Cholesterol: Too much fat in diet. May lead to heart and blood vessel disease.

CL - Chloride: Too much salt. Thirst, water retention and elevated blood pressure.

CO2 Bicarb: Too much protein. Rapid breathing; shortness of breath.

Creat - Creatinine: Inadequate dialysis. Symptoms are nonspecific.

Glu - Glucose: Excessive thirst. Could indicate diabetes.

HBsAG - Hepatitis B Surface Antigen: Fever, malaise, anorexia, nausea, vomiting, urticaria, angioedema and arthritis.

Hct - Hematocrit: Decreased production of red blood cells. Fatigue, shortness of breath, and chest pain on exertion.

154

HIV-1 - Human Immunodeficient Virus:	Persistent cough, malaise and fever.
K - Potassium:	Too much potassium-rich foods. Extreme weakness.
LDH - Lactic dehydrogenase:	Elevation may indicate muscle damage.
Magnesium:	Too much phosphate binders. Decreased mental function.
Na - Sodium:	Too much salt. Thirst, water retention and elevated blood pressure.
Phosphorus:	Too much dairy, organ meats and beans. High and Low: Muscle weakness, continuous bone pain.
P - Potassium:	Too much potassium-rich foods. Weakness, nausea, vomiting. Could lead to cardiac arrest.
SGOT - Serum glutamic oxaloacetic transaminase:	Hepatitis. Nausea, vomiting, abnormal cramping and fatigue.
SGPT:	Hepatitis. Nausea, vomiting, abnormal cramping and fatigue.
T. Bili - Total bilirubin:	Elevation may indicate liver damage or hepatitis.
TP - Total protein:	Best indicator of protein intake.
Trig - Triglycerides:	High level indicates liver damage, hepatitis, or obstruction of bile ducts.
Uric Acid:	High level indicates gout, arthritis, or kidney stones.
WBC - White blood cell count:	High level indicates infection; temperature, chills, nausea, vomiting, and headache. Low level indicates immunosuppression, leukemia; extreme fatigue.

COOK BOOKS FOR RENAL PATIENTS & RECOMMENDED SEASONINGS

"Creative Cooking for Renal Diets" (288 recipes)
"Creative Cooking for Renal Diabetic Diets" (187 recipes)
Send credit card order or check payable to:
SENAY PUBLISHING
P.O. Box 397
Chesterland, Ohio 44026
Cost: $14.95 each
Orders of 6 or more may deduct 25%
Shipping: $2 for one book plus $1 for each additional book
Sales Tax: Ohio residents add $.86 per book

"Living Well on Dialysis"
National Kidney Foundation, Inc.
Council on Renal Failure
30 East 33rd Street
New York, NY 10016
800-622-9010

"The Renal Gourmet"
Send check or money order to:
EMENAR INC.
1545 Lee Street, Suite 6100
Des Plaines, IL 60018
$17.80 + $3.20 S&H = $21.00

"Kidney Cooking"
National Kidney Foundation of
Georgia, Inc.
1655 Tullie Circle, Suite 111
Atlanta, Georgia 30329
Attn: Chuck Brown
Patient Services Mgr.

**60 Days of Low-Fat, Low-Cost
Meals in Minutes**
(Available in bookstores or)
Chronimed Publishing
P.O. Box 59032
Minneapolis, MN 55459-9686

MRS. DASH
Seasoning Blends
(regular grind, table grind)

LOWRY'S
Natural Choice Seasonings

ACCENT
Sodium Free Seasonings

SPICE ISLAND
Salt Free Seasonings

McCORMICK'S
Salt Free Parsley Patch Herb & Spice Blends

ORGAN AND TISSUE DONATION

Because of the advances in transplant surgery, transplantation has made it possible for the blind to see, the crippled to walk, and the very ill to have a better quality of life for thousands of individuals. This is all made possible by the generosity and willingness of individuals or their families to donate organs and tissues. The greater the number of donations, the greater the number of lives that can be saved or improved. You may indicate your wishes to be an organ donor by telling your next of kin, by having a donor symbol on your Florida driver license, and by carrying a donor card.

Organ donors are those individuals who die as a result of severe brain injury. Among the twenty-five organs and tissues, the most commonly transplanted with success are: kidneys, livers, heart/heart valves, lungs, pancreas, corneas/eyes, skin, and bone/bone marrow.

For specific step by step information on recovery centers and transplant programs, or for detailed information on how to become an organ or tissue do nor with the state of Florida contact:

The Nielsen Organ Transplant Foundation or call/write to:

Methodist Medical Center Plaza
580 West Eighth Street
Jacksonville, FL 32209
904-798-8999

Florida Statewide Organ
& Tissue Donor Program
2302 Swann Avenue, Suite B
Tampa, FL 33609
813-251-6488

A complete packet will be provided. This packet will contain answers to many commonly asked questions, additional reading material and a donor card.

NATIONWIDE TELEPHONE NUMBER FOR THE NATIONAL COALITION ON ORGAN AND TISSUE DONATION:
(including recovery centers)
1100 Boulders Parkway, Suite 500, Richmond, VA 23225 - **804-330-8620**
call this number to ask specific questions or to contact your local
Coalition Representative - 800-355-SHARE
call this number to request literature on becoming a donor and
how to speak to your family about this decision.
Web site: www.shareyourlife.org

RECOVERY CENTERS AND
TRANSPLANT PROGRAMS

Central Florida Lion's Eye
Tissue Bank, Inc.,
Tampa FL **(813)977-1300**
800-445-4620

East Central Florida
Transplant Program Florida
Hospital, Orlando
407-894-1390 Nights and
weekends: **407-896-6611**

Florida Lion's Eye Bank
Miami **305-324-4340**
800-255-GIVE

LifeLink of Florida, Tampa
813-253-2640 or 800-64-DONOR
800-822-GIVE

Tallahassee Organ Donor
Agency, Tallahassee
850-877-1150

University of Florida Tissue
Bank, Inc.,
904-392-4251
800-822-GIVE

University of Miami Transplant
Program, Miami **305-547-6315**
800-255-GIVE

Central Florida Tissue Bank, Inc. and
A division of Central Florida
Blood Bank, Inc., Orlando, FL
407-894-6100 or 407-423-4811

Eye Bank Association of America
1001 Connecticut Avenue, N.W.
Suite 601, Washington, DC 20036
202-775-4999
202-429-6030 (fax)

Florida Regional Bone and
Tissue Bank, Inc. Tampa
813-866-8111 or 800-64-DONOR

Medical Eye Lion's Eye Bank,
Inc., Gainesville **904-392-3135**

University of Florida Organ
Procurement Program,
Gainesville **904-392-3711**
800-822-GIVE

University of Miami Tissue
Bank, Miami **305-243-6786**
Nights & weekends, fax:
305-385-1976

APPENDIX - Z
AMERICANS WITH DISABILITIES ACT
OF 1990
Your Rights In The Workplace

"It is the purpose of the Act to provide a clear and comprehensive national mandate for the elimination of discrimination against individuals with disabilities..." -The Americans with Disabilities Act of 1990. Sec. 2(b).

The Americans with Disabilities Act of 1990 was signed by President George Bush on July 26, 1990 and provides job rights for approximately 43,000,000 disabled Americans effective July 26, 1992, for employers of 25 or more employees and (July 26, 1994 for employers of 15 or more employees). The Act compliments the Civil Rights Act of 1964 to now prohibit job discrimination against individuals with disabilities. The ADA includes all employers whether governmental or in the private sector. This also includes employment agencies, labor organizations and joint labor-management committees.

The ADA prohibits pre-employment physicals and pre-employment brain examination but does allow drug testing. The ADA also provides reasonable accommodation for the disabled and empowers the Equal Employment Opportunity Commission (EEOC) to investigate possible violations of the Act. The Act defines a disability as: a physical or mental impairment that substantially limits one or more major life activities; there must be a record of such an impairment; and being regarded as having such an impairment. This definition covers a wide range of individuals including kidney patients.

The ADA says that you cannot discriminate against a qualified individual with a disability in regards to job application procedures, the hiring, advancement, or discharge of employees, employee compensation, and other terms, conditions, and private employment. Reasonable Accommodation basically says that existing facilities must be readily accessible and usable by employees with disabilities. Also, job restructuring, part-time or modified work schedule reassignment to a vacant position must also be provided if necessary. This information is not a substitute for legal advice. It advisable to contact the AAKP or consult with your attorney for further information on the Act or other laws as they apply to your specific case. Public Information System: 1-800-669-EEOE. American Civil Liberties Union, National Headquarters, 132 West 43rd Street, New York, NY 10036 - 212-944-9800.

INDEX

COPYRIGHT
ACKNOWLEDGEMENTS

A WONDERFUL GIFT FOR A KIDNEY PATIENT,
FAMILY MEMBER, FRIEND OR HEALTH CARE PROFESSIONAL
WHO WOULD ENJOY READING SOMETHING INSPIRATIONAL.

ORDER FORM

YES, I want .... copies of Your Kidney/My Kidney, at $19.95 each, plus $3 shipping per book. Canadian orders must be accompanied by a postal money order in U.S. funds. Allow 30 days for delivery.

.... Check or money order enclosed.

Name _____

Phone_____

Address_____

_____

City/State/Zip_____

Check your leading bookstore.
Please make your check payable and return to:

Batax Museum Publishing
2051 Wheeler Lane
Jacksonville, FL 32259

Donna-Marie H. Pollard
Your Kidney/My Kidney